OSTEOPATHIC SELF-TREATMENT

Safe and effective self-help techniques for relaxing tense muscles and easing pain

OSTEOPATHIC SELF-TREATMENT

Safe and effective self-help techniques for relaxing tense
muscles and easing pain

LEON CHAITOW D.O., M.R.O.

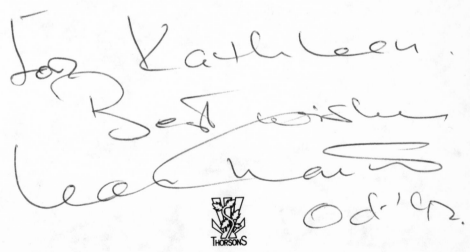

For Kathleen.
Best wishes
Leon Chaitow
Oct '92.

THORSONS

THORSONS PUBLISHING GROUP

First published 1990

© Leon Chaitow 1990

British Library Cataloguing in Publication Data

Chaitow, Leon
Osteopathic self treatment.
1. Man. Musculoskeletal system. Self-treatment
I. Title
616.7'06

ISBN 0-7225-1477-8

Illustrated by Alison Marsh

Published by Thorsons Publishers Limited, Wellingborough, Northamptonshire, NN8 2RQ, England

Typeset by Harper Phototypesetters Limited, Northampton, England
Printed in Great Britain by Mackays of Chatham, Kent

1 3 5 7 9 10 8 6 4 2

Dedication

I would like to affectionately dedicate this book to a host of my American friends within the 'bodywork' community, most specifically to some special caring and nurturing individuals Iris Burman, Sherry Fears, Sandy Cochrane Fritz, Paul Frizzell, Bob and Kathy King, Kerry Ann Plunkett, Cheri Sexton, Carol Simcheck and Charlotte Small, as well as their associates and helpers, and the many hundreds of practitioners and students whom I have had the good fortune to be able to both teach and learn from, over the past few years, through their schools and organization.

Contents

How to use this book

This book describes some common musculoskeletal problems, and shows how these can be alleviated by the use of self-help variations of special osteopathic techniques known as muscle energy technique and strain/counterstrain technique. The book is, however, not intended to be a substitute for professional treatment. The methods explained are, though, very effective and useful in dealing with day-to-day sprains and stiffness, and they are also of considerable value as an augmentation of professional treatment.

Guidance is given on position, timing and frequency, and, in many cases, on breathing and eye movement, so that the choice of the most appropriate action for any particular problem should not be difficult to make.

As a 'rule of thumb', if restriction exists use Muscle Energy Techniques (MET) to produce either post-isometric relaxation or reciprocal inhibition; if weakness exists use isokinetic contraction to tone the muscles; if a large area is weakened, and this can be controlled using appropriate counterpressure, use isotonic techniques. DO NOT, in self-treatment, attempt to use isolytic contractions.

If pain is felt, beyond simple discomfort, whilst using any of the methods described, then stop immediately. If the right technique has been selected, and is properly used, then there will be no pain.

When being used to generally loosen muscles which have become tight, whether through misuse or over-use, MET is safe and effective. But, if you are in any doubt about the applicability of the methods described, or if a condition fails to respond fairly quickly, then seek the advice of a qualified expert, whether this be an osteopath, a chiropractor, a physiotherapist, a licensed massage therapist or a suitably qualified doctor.

Strain/counterstrain techniques can be used to deal with painful recent strains, before, after and instead of muscle energy techniques, and these are described in Chapter 7.

Once the principles of MET and strain/counterstrain have been well understood they can be modified to help most muscle and joint problems.

Introduction

Osteopathic medicine is now over 100 years old and is established in its home country, the USA, as a complete alternative medical discipline, incorporating much of mainstream medicine as well as unique approaches and concepts arising from a deeply held holistic philosophy of health. This views the person as an integrated whole, in which mechanical dysfunction is seen to be capable of influencing the overall health of the individual just as markedly as can other elements such as mento-emotional and nutritional factors.

In Europe and other parts of the world osteopathy has become synonymous with care of musculoskeletal problems and body maintenance. Over the past century the methods and techniques of osteopathy have continued to evolve and develop, until today osteopathic practitioners have at their disposal an array of methods, techniques and systems from which to choose in dealing with the various multiple dysfunctions of the human machine.

Osteopathic health care and body maintenance *always* takes account of causes rather than simply treating the obvious symptoms. Thus a joint problem would be looked at in relation to the other structures of the body and how they influence it, and how it influences them, as well as in terms of the way the person uses and abuses their body in daily use: occupation, sport, postural habits, emotional stresses etc.

All these elements, added to the history of the individual, provide the osteopathic practitioner with a holistic overview of the problem and an understanding of what is required, not only to help the present symptom picture but to prevent recurrence, if this is possible. In therapeutic terms, recent emphasis has been towards a greater appreciation of the importance of the soft tissues in normalizing and easing such problems.

The soft tissues include the muscles, ligaments, fascia, tendons etc. which provide aspects of the supportive matrix which normal bio-mechanical function requires. When joint dysfunction exists initial attention should be given to the soft tissues before attempting to normalize joint function.

The methods which make up the bulk of this book are those which pay particular attention to the soft tissues, and they are in many instances amenable to self-treatment. This, though, is not meant to detract from the benefits available from proper professional attention, and the methods outlined in this book are essentially first-aid and short-term measures which may accompany, precede, or follow regular osteopathic or chiropractic attention. They also can be used for the prevention of problems.

Traditionally, the methods used in osteopathy in order to release and relax tense, tight muscles and joints have involved a variety of manoeuvres in which the tissues have been stroked, stretched, pressed and generally manipulated by the practitioner. In recent years developments have taken place in our understanding of the ways in which the muscles and other soft tissues work, which has brought forth new methods of treatment. Some of these are suitable for adaptation to self-treatment, since they are so safe and gentle that it is almost impossible to cause harm, even if they are performed badly; though obviously their correct performance is more desirable as this will enhance the results.

The methods which form the major focus of this book are pooled together under a general heading of *Muscle Energy Techniques* and what are called functional techniques including *Strain/counterstrain* methods. In addition I will explain a variety of simple measures which can loosely be termed *self-mobilization methods*.

Muscle energy implies that the effort and energy of the individual performing the movements (i.e. the patient) provides the primary force involved in the healing and normalizing process, as distinct from the effort and energy of a practitioner, whether this be an osteopath, chiropractor, masseur, physiotherapist etc.

The conditions which can be helped, and often completely overcome by these methods are myriad, and include a wide range of joint and muscle complaints involving stiffness, restriction of movement, pain and disability. If the problem involves actual pathology, say a condition of arthritis in which destruction of aspects of the joint surface has taken place, then the amount of benefit which might be anticipated would be limited by that damage. Nevertheless, there is no situation, no matter how much damage has occurred, in which the use of appropriate muscle energy methods will not produce some degree of improvement, even if this is not long lasting in all conditions.

Strain/counterstrain methods use newfound osteopathic knowledge of what is termed positional release, in which spasm and contraction associated with injury or strain can be gently 'persuaded' to release by careful positioning of the area or joint, using a local tender area as a guide to the most suitable position for this release. No more gentle method exists for relief of injury, especially if this is of recent origin. Such methods are as suitable for self-help use as muscle energy techniques.

Self-mobilization and exercise are self-explanatory terms. The examples selected for inclusion in this book will be found to offer a variety of means for freeing restricted areas as well as for maintaining freedom once achieved. Prevention is also the aim in many of the examples offered. These methods will be described in greater detail as we progress. Where the primary problem lies in the soft tissues, and does not include actual disease or pathology, the chances are great of achieving, by these methods (especially muscle energy and strain/counterstrain) complete resolution of stiffness and restriction, and often of pain as well.

Referred Pain

In many cases of bodily pain there is an element of referred pain or reflex activity, in which the area of pain is actually some distance from the source of the problem. I will outline the nature of these trigger points and how to find them. A variety of methods have been used in which the 'trigger' points are dealt with and I will explain some of these. See also my book *Instant Pain Control* (Thorsons). The use of muscle energy techniques (MET) provides another excellent way in which these can be either obliterated or minimized.

Variations

MET (Muscle Energy Technique) methods can also be used to strengthen weakened flaccid muscles by a variation in the application of the forces involved. We therefore have in MET a series of methods whereby we may loosen tight muscles and strengthen weak ones. This can be of enormous value in the correction and alleviation of a vast number of painful, stiff and debilitating musculoskeletal problems.

Not all the variations in the use of MET are suitable for self-help methods, since some require the restraining or supporting hands of another person, but a family member or friend can often provide this extra pair of hands. In many situations, of course, an expert is required to control the precise directions and degrees of effort, and so in the text of this book I will attempt to indicate just where self-help is suitable and

where outside aid is necessary.

It should go without saying that these methods should be used only where the cause of the problem is understood, since there is little value in attempting to minimize stiffness and pain if their cause lies in a disease process which is being ignored (see Important Caution, page 51). If attention is being paid to underlying conditions, there are few areas of soft tissue and joint disability and pain, which cannot benefit to some degree from the intelligent use of muscle energy and strain/counterstrain techniques.

Many osteopaths and physiotherapists are now employing these methods which are less uncomfortable for the patient, as well as being less exhausting for the practitioner than many traditional methods. Some of these practitioners are teaching their patients simple home applications, especially of MET, and it is hoped that this handbook will expand that trend. The rules for the successful use of both MET and strain/counterstrain techniques demand an understanding of the basic principles of the physiology involved. There are variations available, and it is wise to know the reasons for their choice.

In the next section I deal with the various types of muscle energy techniques and also have a look at some of the ways in which these work. In a later section I examine a wide range of strain/counterstrain methods for home application.

It is suggested that the reader attempts to understand the whys and wherefores, as explained in the following chapters, before attempting to use any of the individual methods described in later chapters. There is no more certain way of failing to obtain benefits, than by attempting to use wrongly what appears to be a simple method.

The mistakes which are commonest in muscle energy techniques, when applied by the layman, are those which involve **excessive use of force, over too prolonged (or too short) a period of time.** Apart from the **direction in which the effort is made,** these two factors are the most important, and emphasis will be placed on them many times. A central question to ask is, therefore: For how long must an effort be maintained, and with what degree of effort?

These are the key elements in muscle energy technique apart from the overriding importance of the direction of that effort.

- **In none of the methods which will be described in this book should any pain result.**
- **If pain is felt whilst they are being done, stop immediately.**

In no instance should excessive effort be required, and if there is any pain, either the choice of method or the way it is being used is incorrect.

1

The different forms of muscle energy technique

When you bend your elbow, or any other joint, a muscle or group of muscles (known as the agonist(s)) contracts in order to produce movement in the desired direction, whilst at the same time another muscle, or set of muscles (known as the antagonist(s)), relaxes so that the movement will be produced in a smooth co-ordinated manner.

The co-ordination between the opposing muscles of any area is automatic and it happens without conscious effort. It depends upon a physiological law which declares that contraction of one muscle will produce, under normal conditions, relaxation of its antagonist.

When we speak of muscles being antagonistic, we of course do not mean that they have a grudge against their fellows. Rather it indicates that one muscle's action will be directly opposed by another's. They balance each other, and thus work together co-operatively by virtue of the one releasing its contraction, and relaxing, as the other contracts, to produce co-ordinated movement.

Thus, taking the example of the elbow, as the muscles on the front of your arm (the flexors) contract, in order to allow you to lift a glass to your lips, so the muscles on the back of your arm, the extensors, relax, in order to allow this to happen.

The flexors in this example are contract-

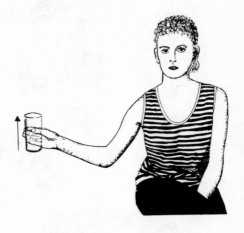

Concentric contraction

ing, and as they do so they are getting shorter. This is called a **concentric contraction**. While this is happening it is, of course, important for the antagonists to continue to exert some effort in order to maintain stability. If they were completely relaxed (e.g. paralysed) then the movement would be uncontrolled, unco-ordinated, spastic and jerky.

When it is time to put the glass down again, the opposite happens. As the extensors straighten out your elbow, the flexors, in a controlled manner, release their hold on your bent joint.

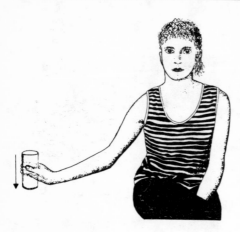

Eccentric contraction

In this particular example, however, the flexors of your arm (which bent it in the first place) do not just release all effort, or there would be sudden straightening of your arm, and the glass would smash onto the table. Rather, they continue to contract, but whilst they are doing so they get longer and release the pull on your elbow. Being able to contract, and at the same time stretch is a most important facility. It is called an **eccentric contraction** and I will return to it later.

It is neccessary to be aware of the fact that muscles are mutually antagonistic to their opposite numbers, and that this offers us a wonderful way of making tight muscles relax. The automatic quality of an antagonist relaxing, when its opposite number is tightening (contracting), is known as **reciprocal inhibition.**

The integrated manner in which the nervous system controls muscular tension, and the importance in this process of

minute reporting stations in the soft tissues, has provided the osteopathic profession with an understanding of the way all this happens. How can we use this knowledge?

If the muscles of the front of your arm, to stay with our first example, are tense, say after gardening, tennis or an injury, you could use the muscles on the back of your arm to relax these tight muscles. If you took that arm to its maximum comfortable degree of straightness, ensuring that in doing so it does not produce pain (which it would if it went beyond its present restrictive barrier), and at that point, whilst restraining your lower arm with your other hand (i.e. preventing it from moving) made an attempt to gently take your arm towards a greater degree of straightness, by contracting the muscles of the back of your arm, what would happen?

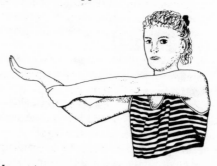

Isometric contraction

Making muscles relax

As you tried to make your arm straight (i.e. pushing gently towards the restrictive barrier) you would be contracting the muscles of the back of your arm. These are the antagonists of the tight muscles which are in trouble. By preventing any movement from taking place (by using your other hand) it is possible to ensure that no strain occurs at the painful joint, or in the tight muscle(s). You would in effect have a matching of forces. The extensor muscles would be trying to pull your arm straight while your free arm resisted this, completely and exactly. This is called an **isometric contraction**. The forces match each other and no movement occurs.

As this isometric contraction of the extensor muscles was taking place in order to try to straighten your arm, their antagonists (the shortened flexors) would be obliged to relax, according to physiological law. Therefore, after this isometric effort, which could last for five to ten seconds, it would be found that the arm which was previously limited in its ability to straighten, would be capable of an increased degree of normality.

The barrier, or point of bind, would have been pushed back a little. By repeating this whole procedure several times until no further gain in the range of movement is noted, it might be possible to completely normalize the shortened muscles.

What I have described above is an example of an **isometric contraction** which is utilizing **reciprocal inhibition**.

There is also another completely different method of doing exactly the same thing. If your arm with a limited ability to straighten was taken as far as it could comfortably go in that direction, (to the current barrier of movement) and this time an attempt was made to *bend* your arm, instead of making it straighter, as in the previous example, and if this effort to bend your arm were resisted by your other hand, you would be doing the

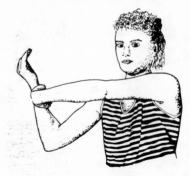

Post-isometric relaxation

opposite of the exercise which produced reciprocal inhibition. Your arm, having been taken to the point of bind would be trying to bend, but the counterforce of your restraining hand would stop it from doing so.

This time, the very muscles which had shortened, after the gardening (or tennis) injury, would be contracting against resistance, and, after an appropriate period, say five to ten seconds, of isometric contraction (no movement allowed to occur, only effort) a new phenomenon would become apparent. This is called **post-isometric relaxation**. This means that any muscle or group of muscles which is isometrically contracted *has to* relax afterwards. So if a muscle is tense or tight, and it is then isometrically contracted, it will, to some extent, release and relax afterwards.

Let us recapitulate. By using the affected muscle(s) in an isometric contraction we induce post-isometric relaxation (PIR). By using the antagonists of affected muscles (tight, shortened etc.) in an isometric contraction we induce reciprocal inhibition

(RI). These are the two keys to the release of troubled muscles and joints using muscle energy methods, and I will be repeating these basic instructions many times during the course of this book.

In some cases, the counterpressure against the contracting muscle(s) will be provided by your own or someone else's hand(s); in other instances it will be provided by an unyielding obstacle, such as a piece of furniture, against which effort can be directed and in yet other cases the counterforce will be gravity.

In all of these, the aim is to use the affected muscles or their antagonists appropriately, in order to achieve the release of tense, tight, shortened muscles, which are often painful, and which usually produce some degree of limitation of movement.

Which method should be used, PIR (post-isometric relaxation), or RI (reciprocal inhibition)?

The presence of pain is frequently used as the deciding factor in choosing one or other of the methods described (PIR or RI). It is clear that when using PIR, the very muscles which have shortened are being contracted. If the condition of the area is one in which there is a good deal of pain, where any contraction could well induce more pain, it might be best to avoid their use and bring into play the antagonists. Thus use of the antagonists, which are usually pain-free, will usually be the first choice in such a muscle energy strategy where the shortened structures are very sensitive. Later, when pain has been reduced by means of muscle energy (or other) methods, PIR techniques

(which use isometric contraction of the already shortened muscles rather than the antagonists used in RI methods) could be used. To a large extent, just how acute or chronic a condition is can help decide the method best suited to treating it, and guidance regarding this will be found later in this chapter.

Thinking back to the example of the arm which is putting down a glass, it may be recalled that muscles can both contract and lengthen at the same time.

Breaking down adhesions and fibrosis

This facility is used in a muscle energy variation called an **isolytic contraction**. When the muscles of your arm were contracting and bringing a glass to your lips, they were both contracting and shortening. Technically this is called a **concentric contraction**. This means that the origins and insertions of the muscle(s) which are contracting, are getting closer together.

In contrast to this, when your arm was putting the glass down, the muscles were contracting, but despite this they were also lengthening. Technically this is known as an **eccentric contraction**. Here the muscle origin and insertion (where the muscle inserts into bone as an anchor point) get further apart, despite the contraction of the muscle.

If muscles have developed a degree of fibrous contraction due to lengthy periods of misuse or injury, (i.e. the condition is chronic), it is often possible to stretch or break down these fibrous structures by means of heavy, deep massage techniques, combined with electrotherapy such as ultrasonic, or other similar methods. However, another method, a muscle energy variation, can also achieve this with far less effort.

If a muscle (or group of muscles) had fibrotically shortened in such a way, and it was actively and vigorously contracted whilst at the same time that contraction was more than matched by counterpressure, and by this means the effort to move in a particular direction was not only matched, but surpassed, then the area would be **eccentrically contracting**. The muscles would be trying to move a joint in one direction but the counterpressure would force it in the opposite direction. The origin and insertion of this muscle would be attempting to come closer together, but the counterforce inducing the isolytic contraction would force them apart.

An example of this could be of contraction in the muscles of your hand or palm, which prevented your fingers from opening fully. Were there an effort to make your hand close, at the same time as an effort to overcome this were being made by your other hand, which would be grasping your fingers, and which actually forced the other hand further open against its attempted closing effort, then an eccentric contraction would have occurred in the flexors of the hand or fingers.

This would be called an isolytic contraction and the exercise would have broken down some of the fibrous adhesions in the muscles of that hand. **This use of muscle energy methods can be painful and is not suggested as a home therapy, unless directed by a practitioner.** It is described only in order to comprehensively present muscle energy methods.

Toning weak muscles

A further variation exists in which the muscle which is being contracted is resisted, but not fully. This results in an **isotonic contraction**.

Let me explain. Recall that in PIR and RI we have equal and opposite forces involved (the muscle's own effort and a counterpressure which matches this) which are producing *isometric* contractions and resulting in release of tightness.

In *isolytic* contractions we have a contracting force which is not just matched but which is actually overcome by the counterpressure.

In *isotonic* contractions we have a contraction which is matched, but not quite overcome. The movement is allowed to take place, but against resistance. Should a group of muscles be weak, after disuse for example, and should you wish to tone these up, you have a perfect tool in isotonic methods of muscle energy.

Now let us assume that the flexors (which bend your elbow) of your arm are weak, for whatever reason. If your opposite hand were placed on your forearm to partially restrain an attempt to bend your arm then, as they contracted, the weak muscles would be working against a degree of resistance. By repeatedly doing this, with variations in the degree of resistance applied, it would be possible to rapidly retrain the weak muscles to a degree of normality.

This would be called an **isotonic con-**

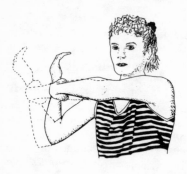

Isotonic concentric contraction

centric contraction. Were it possible to rapidly and repeatedly move a particular area in a variety of directions, all the while partially restraining these with the other hand, then the description of this manoeuvre would be an **isokinetic contraction**.

An example of this could involve a weak ankle, in which it is possible, by sitting with the affected leg resting across the other knee, to use the hands to restrain a forceful effort to put the ankle joint through as full a range of movements as possible, in a short space of time (no more than five seconds). This has a powerful toning effect on the whole joint. This isotonic series of movements would be an example of isokinetic muscle energy technique.

The major variables in MET

As in all the examples given, the essence of the methods is the amount of effort used in restraining a contraction, as well as the amount of effort used in that contraction. The other major variables which are controllable are, of course, how long the contraction is allowed to continue, and how often it is repeated. The degree of effort in isometric contractions is *always* much less than the full force available from the muscles involved. The initial contraction should involve the use of a quarter or less of the strength available. This, of course, will not be an exact measurement, but indicates that we do not ever want a wrestling match to develop between the contracting area and the counterforce, whether this be a hand, a piece of furniture, another person's hands, or gravity.

After the initial contraction, subsequent contractions may involve an increase in effort, but should never reach more than half of the full strength of that muscle. We want above all to achieve a *controlled* degree of effort at all times, and this calls for the use of only part of the latent strength in a muscle or muscle group.

However, when we are using isolytic contractions in which the contraction is overcome by a counterforce, then the degree of effort used in the contraction should be fairly strong, often the full strength of the muscle.

(This particular method is *not* a home treatment technique as a rule, and the practitioner employing these methods would control the range, direction and timing of the effort(s), which normally involve shorter periods of contraction (often only 2 to 4 seconds)).

The timing of isometric contractions is usually such as to allow at least five, and up to ten, seconds for the contraction, from beginning to end.

It is important to remember that the start and the end of contraction should always be slow. There should never be a snatching, or a quick beginning or end to the contraction. Always attempt a smooth build-up of power in the muscle(s) and a slow switch-off of the contraction at the end. This will prevent injury or strain, and allows for the best possible results.

In some cases it will be found that slightly shorter periods of time are suggested for the contractions, and in others they will be longer. Indeed, in many instances there is a variation as the therapy progresses, with even longer periods of time involved, although 30 seconds would be a top limit, unless otherwise stated in the text. **It is far safer and more effective to contract a muscle for a longer period than it is to make the contraction stronger.**

Guidance as to these variables will be given in the individual examples later in the book. As a rough guide, though, the 5–10 second timing of initial isometric contractions is a useful rule to have in mind. Repetitions are normally continued three or four times, although usually only for as long as improvements continue to be achieved in the problem muscle(s) between contractions.

A practical example of PIR

As an example, let us return to the arm which is difficult to straighten fully. Let us say this is the right arm. The first objective is always to engage the restrictive barrier. This arm will not easily straighten, so it should therefore be taken gently to the limit of the available degree of movement, in the direction in which it is restricted. Going too far would force it beyond the current barrier, and would actually irritate the tissues of the area, so it should therefore be stretched out gently, until the 'point of bind' is felt, beyond which discomfort would start. If you are trying to release and stretch tissues which are chronically short (this usually means they have been that way for a month or more) then the isometric contraction should start some way short of the restrictive barrier, or 'point of bind'. If the condition is acute (less than a month old) the contraction should start at the restrictive barrier. The degree of effort used in acute and chronic conditions also varies as you will see below.

Sitting at a table the right arm could be rested on it, as straight as it is comfortably possible to do, and the left hand placed at about wrist level in order to restrain a contraction of the muscles which bend the arm (the very ones which have shortened and which prevent full straightening). As the attempt was being made to bend the arm, the counterpressure from the left hand would be preventing this. Only about a quarter of the available force in the muscles of the right arm is used, and the onset of the contraction is synchronised with the counterpressure so as to avoid any jerking. This contraction would then be maintained for a slow count of 10 before being slowly released, in a co-ordinated manner, together with the release of the counterpressure from the left hand.

After a moment in which the arm is relaxed fully, (a breathing technique can be used to enhance this, see below), an attempt should be made to take the arm to its fullest, pain-free, stretched-out length. This stretch should push just beyond the restrictive barrier if the condition is chronic (an old problem, of more than a month's duration) and just to the barrier if it is acute (a more recent problem). Thus the new barrier would be engaged and there should be noted a slightly greater degree of movement than was possible before the isometric contraction. The arm can now be taken a little straighter without effort.

When this new limit of straightness is reached, the whole procedure is repeated again, exactly as above, except that if the condition has existed for a month or more the length of the resisted contraction could be longer, going up to 15 seconds. There could also be a slight increase in the degree of effort employed. If the condition is acute the same mild (no more than 25 per cent of available strength) contraction is used for repetitions. Then again, after co-ordinated release of the contraction and the counterpressure, another attempt could be made to see just how straight the arm could go, painlessly.

When, after two or three repetitions of the isometric contraction no further gain is noted in terms of increased stretching ability in the shortened muscles, (i.e. the barrier of movement remains the same before and after an isometric contraction), then enough would have been done for one day, by use of post isometric relaxation, on the contracted tissues.

Use of RI

It would then be appropriate to attempt to gain a little more ease of movement by using the reciprocal inhibition method, in which the antagonists are employed. Reciprocal inhibition is often more useful in acute conditions.

To do this, the arm should again be taken to its full comfortable resting length, with the elbow on the table, and this time the left hand is placed on the back of the wrist, as a counterforce. This time the effort would involve the extensor muscles, which would try to force the arm into a greater degree of straightness, against resistance from the other hand. Again only partial strength is used, and the timing is the same as above, starting with a 5–10 second contraction.

After a slow easing of the dual efforts, (the arm trying to straighten against resistance), the arm would again be tested to see if it could achieve a greater degree of normality.

Several attempts of this type should be made, increasing the length, and degree, of effort (always ensuring that no pain is produced, and only increasing the amount of muscular effort if the condition is chronic), until it becomes evident that no further gains could be made at that time and it is at this point that muscle energy methods should be stopped for the day. Both PIR and RI would have been used, and maximum gains enjoyed in terms of greater degree of movement and lessened discomfort.

Variations in the direction of the contraction are possible during these various isometric efforts, in which different angles of bending or straightening are resisted, thus using different muscle fibres. For example, the hand of the arm resting on the table could be aiming for the face, as the contraction begins, or it could be aiming for the right or left shoulder.

These variations in direction are always possible when trying to normalize tight muscles, and should be incorporated into the variables of amount of effort used, amount of time of each contraction, number of contractions and type of contraction (PIR or RI).

Other variables in the previous example could include the position of the hand on the affected side during the contractions. This could be palm downwards, or palm upwards, thus bringing into play different muscles. All such factors will be outlined as appropriate, in the descriptions of the various muscles and joints in the text.

Influence of breathing on MET

There is still one more factor relating to these methods which has not been elaborated on up to now, and this involves the use of breathing patterns to enhance the effects of PIR and RI.

In some cases it is necessary to breathe in deeply at the onset of a contraction and to hold the breath for the duration of the effort, releasing the breath at completion, as relaxation is taking place. In other instances it is desirable for the breath to be sighed out as the effort commences, and for this to be held out until the end of the contraction.

In all cases it is desirable that after the contraction, and before any attempt is made to assess the degree of extra movement achieved, a deep breath be taken and sighed out, in order to fully release all muscular effort.

The reasons for the suggested breathing patterns during isometric and isotonic contractions is that there is evidence that certain muscle movements are enhanced by one or other phase of the breathing cycle. For example, if you bend towards your toes whilst breathing in, you will not be able to reach as far as if the same movement were made whilst you were breathing out. This apparently holds true for many other movements of the body as well.

Bending the neck forward, or general sidebending, are two examples of this. The neck and lumbar spine are easier to bend backwards as you breathe out, whereas the thoracic spine is easier to bend backwards when the breath is being taken in. For instance, a bending forwards of the thoracic spine (where the ribs attach) is facilitated by breathing out, whereas the precise reverse is true if this area is being bent backwards.

There is therefore an advantage to be gained in combining the breathing phase most desirable in any given movement, with that movement, or with contraction in that direction. (Guides to these will be given in the text.)

Eye movements and MET

If you try to bend forwards whilst at the same time looking upwards, (with the eyes only, not any movement of the head), you will not bend as far or as easily as if you were looking downwards at such a time. Similarly, the converse applies to coming upright from a bent position with the eyes looking downwards. So, bend forwards with the eyes down and the movement becomes easier, and straighten up from such a bend, or actually bend backwards, with the eyes rolled upwards, and here too the movement becomes easier.

The same eye involvement is noted in other movements as well. Sit in a chair and twist your trunk and head to one side, whilst your eyes are looking in the opposite direction, and try and note just how far you can go without undue strain. Mentally mark a point on the wall as indicating your furthest point of rotation, then do the same turn exactly, but this time have the eyes travelling in the same direction as the twist. You will find that you can go much further because the rotation of the body is improved by the direction in which the eyes are looking. (Guidelines to these variables will be found in the text.)

To sum up, intensity of contraction, direction of contraction, duration of contraction and frequency of contraction are all important factors in successful application of muscle energy methods. Whether to use the affected muscles or their antagonists are fundamental decisions (pain will help to decide this). Breathing and eye movement are peripheral, but useful, refinements which can make the techniques more successful.

This, then, is the essence of Muscle Energy Technique. It is simple, and yet the rules are important, since too much effort or wrong timing will negate the results. But follow the rules closely, and the results will be the best that can be hoped for in any given condition.

These methods do not replace other methods of self-help, and should be combined with whatever else is found helpful, whether this involves self-mobilisation, exercise, self-massage, or any other treatment. MET methods are very useful in preparing a joint for subsequent manipulation, making treatment easier and more effective.

MET techniques are highly desirable as home therapy, since little if any harm can ever come from their use, even when wrongly applied (except for excessive force being exerted). They should never cause pain, and this should be a guide to their use. Pain means that too much effort, or an inappropriate method of muscle energy technique is being used.

These methods can be used daily or several times daily if helpful, or only when necessary and can safely be employed where joints are damaged, as in arthritic conditions, because they will not involve movement of the joints, and can therefore enhance the muscular status, either by releasing tight muscles or toning weak muscles.

There is no single joint or muscle problem which cannot be helped, to some extent, by appropriate muscle energy technique, and in many instances, where the causes involve strain or injury, the results are almost instantaneous and permanent. Spasm, contraction, tightness, stiffness and shortening of muscles represents major causes of pain and disability, and Muscle Energy methods can reduce this and lead to greater freedom of movement and relief of pain in many cases.

2

Explanations and Summary of MET methods

In this section I will summarize and explain some of the variations discussed in the last chapter. I will also attempt to explain just how the subsequent illustrated sections of individual MET methods should be used.

What is an isometric contraction?

This is a contraction in which the effort of the muscle, or group of muscles, is exactly matched by the counterpressure, so that no movement occurs, only effort.

What is an isotonic contraction?

An isotonic contraction is one in which the effort of the muscle, or group of muscles, is not quite matched by the counterpressure, allowing a degree of resisted movement to occur.

What is an isolytic contraction?

An isolytic contraction is one in which the effort of the contracting muscle(s) is more than matched by the counterpressure, and which therefore causes the contracting muscle(s) to be forcibly stretched. An isolytic contraction is a variation of an isotonic contraction.

What is an isokinetic contraction?

An isokinetic contraction involves the movement of a joint through a full range of motion, rapidly, and using full muscle strength, against partial resistance. This is therefore a multiple isotonic movement.

What are the different forms of MET using isometric contraction?

When the actual muscles which have shortened are contracted isometrically, then the phenomenon of *post isometric relaxation* will induce these shortened muscles to relax after the effort. When the antagonists are used in the contraction, the phenomenon of *reciprocal inhibition* will induce the shortened muscles to relax after the effort.

Which of these methods should be chosen?

Either or both may be used, and the only reason for choosing reciprocal inhibition as a starting method would be because of pain or spasm in the region, which could be aggravated by contraction of the already troubled muscles. This would not always occur, but if the pain is acute, or there is great spasm, then RI is suggested before PIR methods.

How do these methods work?

Reciprocal inhibition obliges a muscle to relax because of the increased tone in its antagonist.

This works through the mediation of the central nervous system which cannot allow both the agonist muscle (the prime mover in any given instance) and its antagonist, to both be tightening at the same time (this would lead to movements such as occur in spastic conditions). *Post isometric relaxation* which occurs after an isometric contraction of a muscle, results from the activity of minute neural reporting stations called the golgi tendon bodies. These lie near the origins and insertions of the muscles, and report to the central nervous system (CNS) the load the muscle is having to bear. An isometric contraction, maintained for some seconds, results in a report to the CNS asking for the muscle to be released and relaxed due to excessive load.

It is in the brief latent period of ten seconds or so after such a contraction that the muscle can be stretched painlessly, further than it could before the contraction. Both reciprocal inhibition and post isometric relaxation therefore result from physiological laws being applied, not from force.

What is counterpressure?

Counterpressure is the force applied to an area which is designed to match exactly (isometric contraction) or partially (isotonic contraction) or to overcome (isolytic contraction) the effort, or force, produced by the muscles of that area.

This counterpressure, or holding force, can be applied via the hand(s) of the person doing the exercise, someone else's hands, an immovable object against which pressure can be applied, or against gravity, where this is appropriate.

How can gravity be used as counterpressure?

If the head is hanging over the edge of a bed or table, when you are lying on your side, for example, then a degree of stretch would be being applied to the supporting muscles on the uppermost side of the neck. Gravity would be pulling the head towards the floor, and the restraining muscles would be holding the head, and would be under a good deal of tension.

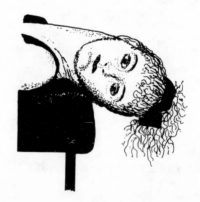

If at that time the head were very slightly lifted by these tense muscles, so that it came towards the midline (i.e. away from the floor) by about a centimetre or so, and if this new position were held, then an isometric contraction would be taking place, in which the contracted muscle's effort would be matched precisely by the pull of gravity against it.

If this position were held for some seconds, together with appropriate breathing patterns, and then slowly released, these muscles would demonstrate post isometric relaxation. And, had they previously been shortened or contracted, then they would now be looser.

This is an example of gravity-induced PIR, and other examples will be found in the text.

How can an immovable object be used as a counterpressure source?

If the muscles on the back of the thigh were shortened, it would be difficult to use the person's own hands, or gravity, to act as counterpressure to their contraction. This could be achieved by placing the foot of the outstretched leg onto a bench or stool, using this as a fixed point against which to apply pressure. By placing the foot on a bench which serves as a resistance to an isometric contraction of the muscles of the back of the leg, a successful isometric contraction can be achieved. The leg would be outstretched and braced against the bench, and by leaning forward a great deal of additional stretch can be localized in these muscles.

Maintaining such a position for an appropriate length of time would produce PIR in them, allowing them to be stretched further after the isometric contraction ceases.

How much force should be generated by the muscles contracting when isometric and other MET methods are used?

With most isometric contractions this should start at about 25 per cent of the strength of the muscle for the first contraction. Subsequent contractions in chronic conditions (more than a month's duration) could involve progressively greater degrees of effort, but *never more* than 50 per cent of the available strength. Many experts use only about 10 per cent of the available strength in muscles being treated in this way, and find that they can increase effectiveness by employing longer periods of contraction. In acute conditions only light contractions are used, starting at the restriction barrier and moving to the new barrier afterwards, unlike the method applied to chronic conditions where the contraction starts short of the barrier and stretches slightly through it afterwards.

In isotonic contractions greater effort may be employed, especially if isokinetic measures are involved, in which case full strength is used. In isolytic contractions only a minimal amount of effort is used at first, progressively building to about half the full muscle strength in subsequent contractions. Contractions and counterpressure should never become a struggle. Always maintain a controlled degree of effort in all such manoeuvres.

How long should the Muscle Energy contractions last?

Isometric contractions should last from 5-10 seconds at first. Subsequent contractions can be progressively longer, but not exceeding half a minute.

Isotonic contractions are usually accomplished in 4–7 seconds, whilst isokinetic contractions should take no more than 4–5 seconds.

How often should contractions be repeated at any one session?

Not less than three times and up to seven or eight is common. With isometric contractions, these are ceased when no further objective improvement is noted in the range of movement of the shortened or tight muscles. However, isokinetic contractions are usually limited to 2 or 3 efforts at any one time.

How regularly should Muscle Energy contractions be used?

Daily if desired, and if no pain is noted. However, in chronic cases regular employment of these methods is suggested until normalization is achieved. This could mean daily, or on alternative days, for many weeks.

Which MET method is best for problems?

Isometric contractions, both those designed to induce post-isometric relaxation and reciprocal inhibition, are best used in dealing with muscular spasm, stiffness, contraction and shortening of muscles. They are also useful in loosening stiff joints, whatever the cause might be. However, the degree of improvement possible in such cases will depend upon the degree of

permanent damage in a joint.

PIR and RI are useful in preparing a joint for subsequent manipulation. The achieving of a muscle's full resting length, after it has been shortened or contracted for any reason, is important in eliminating trigger points which lie in such muscles, and which might be causing pain and other symptoms elsewhere in the body. (See Chapter 5.)

Isotonic concentric contractions are used for toning weakened musculature. Isotonic eccentric contractions (isolytic) are used for stretching and breaking down fibrotic bands in tight muscles. Lastly, isokinetic contractions are used for toning weakened musculature and building strength in all the muscles involved in a particular joint's function.

How long do the effects of relaxation in the tight muscles last?

Tests in Sweden have demonstrated that just one short isometric contraction produced increases in the range of movement in hip and ankle joints of over 15 per cent, which were still measurable some hours after the contraction.

In clinical practice it is found that, once relaxed, a tight muscle will not tighten up again unless provoked or irritated in some manner. Therefore, it is suggested that normal use be resumed after muscle energy measures, but that any violent or potentially irritating exercises be avoided for a few days. The beneficial effects should be permanent, if no reinjury is sustained.

How should the isometric effort be commenced?

In acute conditions, having engaged the barrier (see below) the counterpressure is applied and the contraction commences, slowly.

There should be a build-up of muscular effort, coinciding with the counterpressure, and also coinciding with a breathing pattern which is suitable to that movement. The slow commencement of the effort prevents any jerking or sudden movement, which would ruin the strategy of inducing relaxation in the affected musculature. In chronic conditions, since the contraction used is often stronger than that suggested in acute conditions, this should start short of the barrier to reduce the slight chance of cramp.

How should the isometric effort cease?

The same slow easing of effort is desirable at the end of the effort. After this a deep breath is taken and sighed out slowly, as the muscles of the area involved are consciously relaxed. At this point, the barrier is again tested, in acute conditions, whereas in chronic states a *very slight* stretch is made just beyond the restriction barrier, in order to introduce elasticity into fibrous, shortened tissues.

What is the 'barrier'?

When a joint is restricted or a muscle shortened, thus reducing the range of motion of its associated joint or region, then there will always be a direction in which movement is limited. As the limit of movement, in that restricted direction, is reached, there will be noticed a 'point of bind', beyond which no more comfortable movement is possible.

When a *normal* joint is taken to its limit, it will usually be found that at the end of the range there is still a bit more movement available, a sort of springiness, in the joint. When there is *abnormal* restriction, however, the limit does not have this spring, but rather, as with a jammed door or drawer, it is fixed at that point, and any attempt to take it further is uncomfortable and the feel is distinctly of 'bind' or jamming, rather than springiness. This is the barrier through which muscle energy methods will attempt to take the joint or area, by inducing relaxation in the muscles which are holding it fixed.

This 'end point', or barrier, can be described as having either a 'soft' or 'hard' end-feeling. Soft tissue restrictions always have a softer end-feel than internal joint restrictions which have a sudden, or hard, end-feel.

Are all joint problems the result of such muscle shortening?

By no means, although if there are other reasons such as joint damage or cartilage or tendon injury, the muscles will be involved to some extent, since they are the prime movers of the bones.

Thus, even if other causes than muscle problems are active, the application of MET methods will to some degree be helpful, even if only to a limited degree and for a short time. However, where muscles are the major cause, and this is in the majority of cases, the condition can often be normalized by MET alone.

Where does the breathing and eye movement pattern come into all this?

The use of co-ordinated breathing to enhance particular directions of muscular effort will be outlined where appropriate. As a general rule, all muscular effort is enhanced by breathing in as the effort is made, although in some cases breathing out at such times will be suggested, because of the direction of the effort.

Follow the guidelines where possible, as they will enhance the results, although even without them the result should be satisfactory. The same applies to eye movements.

Summary of PIR or RI MET methods.

1. Choose the type of MET method according to guidelines above.
2. Take the restricted area or joint to its comfortable limit, i.e. engage the barrier. In chronic conditions back off from the barrier before starting the contraction. In acute conditions start at the barrier.
3. Ensure the correct type and placement of counterpressure.
4. Commence contraction and counterpressure simultaneously, breathing as directed, or if no directions are given then breathe in as effort commences. Never use more than 25 per cent of strength unless otherwise instructed.

5. Hold breath in (or out if so directed) and the contraction and counterpressure for the appropriate time (guidelines given), which is usually 5-10 seconds.
6. Ease off both effort and counterpressure in a slow co-ordinated manner as the breath is released (if it has been held), or taken in (if it has been held out).
7. Breathe in deeply, and sigh out slowly, as the muscles are consciously let go.
8. Slowly and carefully re-engage the barrier to assess increased range of movement, in acute conditions, whereas in chronic states go to a point just beyond the barrier to stretch the tight muscle(s) - holding this for 5 to 10 seconds.
9. Never, under any circumstances, forcibly stretch the shortened muscle(s) to the point where pain is produced (mild discomfort is acceptable), as this can produce a reflex reaction, contracting them again.
10. Repeat the whole process several more times, with increased degree of effort and longer periods of contraction, never exceeding half a minute.
11. If no more improvement is noted, cease this type of MET and try the other, (i.e. if PIR has been used try RI, or vice versa).
12. Variations in angle of effort can be used to involve a greater number of muscle fibres, with possible benefit.

Summary of isotonic toning contraction

1. Place counterpressure hand(s) in position and contract the weak muscle forcibly, whilst the counterpressure just fails to control the movement thus induced.
2. Although it is permissible for the full

force of the muscle involved to be utilized in isotonic toning manoeuvres, the start of the contraction should be a slow build-up of force, not a snatching jerk. The action should become one involving maximum muscle effort and the movement achieved should be less than fast, as the counter-pressure allows movement to take place.
3. Effort and counterpressure should cease simultaneously.
4. Repeat 3 or 4 times.

Summary of isolytic contraction

1. The appropriate muscle is placed in maximum stretch and counterpressure applied.
2. A slow application of less than maximum effort in that muscle is commenced, at the same time as the counterpressure, which in this case overcomes the contraction to further forcibly stretch the shortened muscle, breaking down adhesions etc.
3. This may be repeated several times, increasing the degree of contraction if pain is not too great.

Summary of isokinetic contraction

1. Hold the affected joint with one or both hands.
2. Forcibly, and with maximum available effort of the muscles of the joint, attempt to move the joint through its full range of movements, whilst restricting this by counterpressure to an extent, but not fully.
3. Only 3 to 4 seconds is needed at any one time for this to be effective.
4. Repeat several times.

3

Muscles: Types and Tests

Different muscles in the body have, not unnaturally, different roles to play. What is not widely realized is that there are two basically different types of muscles in the body, and that these react differently to stress and strain, and also have quite different functions. These two kinds of muscles can be called types 1 and 2.

Type 1 muscles are concerned with stamina and endurance functions. Their work relates in large part to static, postural or antigravity tasks, requiring long periods of contraction and little speed of action.

Type 2 muscles are those mainly involved in activity, power and speed, and which have, unlike type 1 muscles, little ability to perform tasks of endurance.

The ways in which these different muscles derive their energy is not the same, and neither is the way in which they react to being overused, underused or abused. The static type 1 muscles, which have a primary role in long-term endurance and postural work, will shorten and tighten in response to dysfunction or abuse. The so-called phasic type 2 muscles, which are primarily involved in movement, become weak in response to dysfunction or abuse.

Which problem should be tackled first, weak or tight muscles?

It is commonly held that the first priority in postural correction, or the regaining of fitness, should be the strengthening and toning of weak muscles. This is incorrect.

The fact is that by freeing and loosening tight muscles increased strength in the weak muscles will be automatically achieved. If the muscles of the body are in a general state of unfitness and stiffness, some will be weak and others tight. Therefore to begin a programme aimed at improving function with the toning up of the weak muscles is a mistake. The correct sequence should be to loosen the tight muscles, which then allows a natural regeneration of tone and strength to take place in the weak muscles.

After tightness in the postural muscles has been dealt with, a period of several weeks should elapse before commencing any attempt at toning weak muscles, either by exercise or MET isotonic methods, since many of these will automatically strengthen, once related tightness (i.e. shortening etc.) has been dealt with. This is because of a phenomenon which I have already discussed briefly, reciprocal inhibition.

In the chapters dealing with Muscle Energy Techniques it can be seen that if a muscle (or group of muscles) is contracted, the antagonist(s) will relax and weaken, thus allowing us to gently stretch the tight muscle, had it been short. This highlights the physiological law which states that if a muscle weakens, its antagonist tightens, ànd conversely, if a muscle tightens, its antagonist weakens.

When we have weak muscles in the body there is an automatic shortening, tightening or contracting of the antagonist(s). If we treat these using Muscle Energy Techniques or any other method, and relax and stretch them, then the weak antagonists *have to* strengthen. Muscle Energy Techniques are superbly designed to assist in the freeing and relaxing of tight muscles, (which are most often the type 1 muscles), and any weakness which is found to remain in type 2 muscles, after this has been achieved, can be further treated by using isotonic muscle energy methods, as well as exercises.

This is the correct sequence, since any attempt to tone weak muscles prior to relaxing and loosening tight muscles will have a contradictory effect.

The already tight muscles will become tighter as you attempt to strengthen weak muscles (their antagonists), even if they are not being singled out for toning activity, since there is hardly any exercise involving weak muscles which will not also strengthen and shorten overactive muscles (their antagonists) at the same time. There will in consequence be more dysfunction (pain, stiffness etc.) than if the tight muscles were dealt with first, and released.

An example of this might be of an individual with a large protruding abdomen and a general slouching posture, including a depressed rib cage and rounded shoulders. A common practice in such individuals, before our newfound knowledge of postural and phasic muscles and their different responses to misuse, was to approach such a case by suggesting abdominal toning exercises. This assumed from the outset that the abdominal muscles were weak, since they could not hold the abdomen in, as they should. Palpation of the abdominal muscles in most such people would show, perhaps surprisingly, that far from being weak, these muscles are heroically attempting to hold their burden in place and are in fact tense and tight, especially if the condition is a longstanding one.

If in such a case, MET or other releasing methods were applied to the areas of the neck, shoulders, chest and diaphragm as well as to the postural muscles of the back, at the same time as specific efforts were made to release tension in the overtaxed abdominal muscles, an improvement in overall posture would become apparent. The chest cage, instead of being depressed and held down by tight muscles, would become freer and would be held more correctly, allowing the abdominal muscles to perform their task more easily.

The correction of the protruding abdomen does not lie in *toning* these overworked muscles, but in *releasing* them from the tethered position in which the slouching posture is holding them. If they are indeed weak their antagonists, such as the low back muscles alongside the spine (erector spinae) should be relaxed and stretched as this will usually allow increased tone to return to the abdominal muscles, quite automatically.

MET can do this effectively, as can other methods of soft tissue manipulation, without undue emphasis on exercise. The methods outlined in the book will help in normalizing tight muscles, which we should by now realize have mainly postural roles to play in the body.

Type 1 (postural or endurance) muscles

Among the more important of the postural (type 1) muscles, which become shortened in response to disuse or stress, are the following: Trapezius, sterno-cleido mastoid, levator scapulae, upper fibres of pectoralis major, quadratus lumborum, sacrospinalis (erector spinae), oblique abdominals, iliopsoas, tensor fascia lata, rectus femoris, biceps femoris, semi-tendinosus and semimembranosus (these last three are commonly grouped together as the 'hamstrings'), adductors of the leg (longus, brevis and magnus), piriformis, soleus and tibialis posterior, and the flexor muscles of the arms.

These will be the muscles which are deserving of special attention in terms of stretching and freeing, via Muscle Energy Techniques.

Type 2 (phasic) muscles

Those muscles which are largely phasic (they move the parts of the body but have no great stamina) and which are subject to weakening rather than tightening include: Scaleni, paravertebral cervical muscles, extensors of the arm, abdominal aspects of pectoralis major, middle and inferior branches of trapezius, rhomboids, serratus anterior, rectus abdominus, internal and external obliques, gluteal muscles, vastus (intermedius, lateralis and medialis) and the muscles of lower leg, peroneus brevis and longus, as well as tibialis anticus.

These certainly may at times require relaxing via MET, but are more likely to require toning up, by use of isotonic manoeuvres.

Any muscle of either type 1 or 2 can become strained, and thus shortened as a result of injury or wrong use.

The division into these two muscle types indicates the primary roles which these muscles play and also the basic tendency towards either tightness or weakness, which is inherent in their make-up. It is possible however for a type 1 muscle to become weak and for a type 2 muscle to become tight. It is therefore important to know how to test a muscle to know whether it is either tight or weak.

This really requires an expert assessment, especially in terms of muscle weakness. It is possible however to give general guidelines as to what is more or less normal, and to judge from this whether a degree of tightness is evident in particular muscles. It is important to remember that not all muscles are amenable to self-assessment and some of the tests described below call for help from a friend or member of the family.

The simplest method of identifying the need for MET

In deciding how to self-treat a tight muscle or group of muscles or a stiff joint, there is

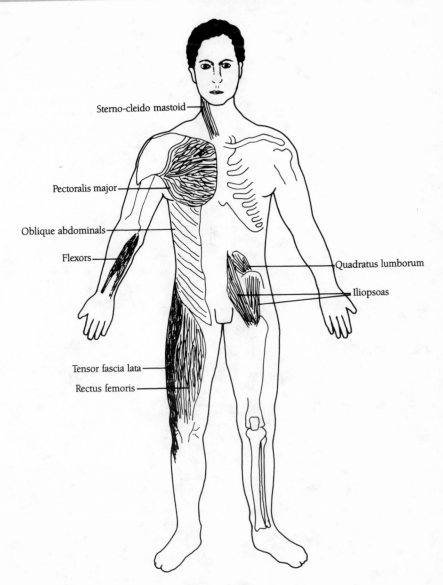

Sterno-cleido mastoid

Pectoralis major

Oblique abdominals

Flexors

Quadratus lumborum

Iliopsoas

Tensor fascia lata

Rectus femoris

Type 1 Postural or endurance muscles

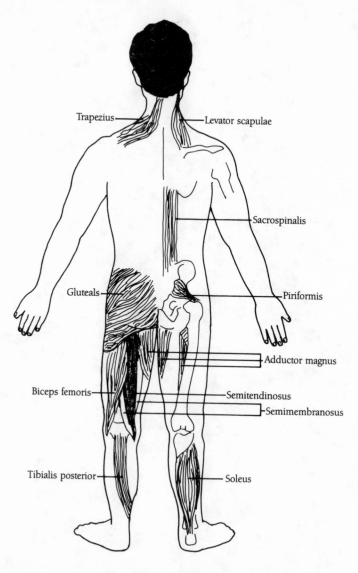

Type 1 Postural or endurance muscles

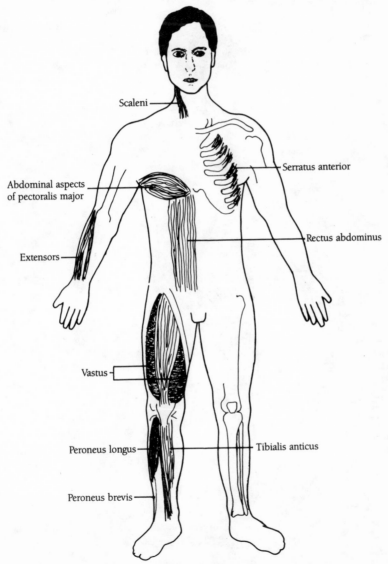

Scaleni

Serratus anterior

Abdominal aspects
of pectoralis major

Rectus abdominus

Extensors

Vastus

Peroneus longus

Tibialis anticus

Peroneus brevis

Type 2 Phasic muscles

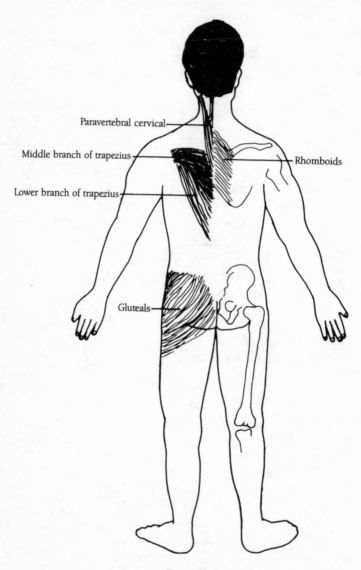

Paravertebral cervical

Middle branch of trapezius

Rhomboids

Lower branch of trapezius

Gluteals

Type 2 Phasic muscles

always a most obvious method which does not depend upon tests of particular muscles, and where restrictions are easily recognisable and which thereby dictate the course of action. If, for example, a knee, an elbow or a finger, (or any other joint) is limited in any of its normal ranges of motion, it will be obvious. By comparison with what is normal or by comparison with what the other fingers, or knee or elbow can do, anyone will be able to know that there is restriction and be able to identify the direction(s) of the restriction.

This is all that is needed to begin MET. If, as an example, the knee cannot bend fully, (indicating shortness of the muscles at the front of the leg), then it should be bent to its pain-free limit and one or other of the isometric MET methods should then be employed. (PIR or RI.)

By restraining the knee with the hands or an immovable object, the bent joint should be made to try to bend further. This uses the antagonists and thus induces reciprocal inhibition, which will tend to release the tense muscles which are preventing the knee from bending. Alternatively, the knee, having been bent to its pain-free limit should be prevented from straightening. This would involve employing the very muscles which are tight, and which are preventing bending of the knee and would produce post isometric relaxation in these shortened muscles, thus helping to normalize them.

The nature and degree of the restriction determines the self-treatment. Either the antagonists or the involved muscles themselves are used, producing either RI or PIR respectively. This same method could be applied to any joint restriction, without any knowledge as to which muscles are involved. Either the restricted joint is forced by its own controlling muscles *towards* the restrictive barrier, or *away from* the barrier, and in each case no movement is allowed, only an isometric contraction. Hence, if the effort of the muscles is towards the barrier, then RI of the shortened muscles will result, and if the effort is away from the barrier then PIR of the shortened muscles will result.

Both efforts will subsequently increase the range of free movement available. The only test necessary is to decide how much improvement has been gained after each isometric contraction has been released and appropriate relaxation achieved, as the joint is taken to its new barrier prior to repeating the exercise.

A stiff neck, restricted low back etc, all call for similar action, and if the methods are applied as directed, then nothing but benefit can be achieved, for no undue effort or strain will be applied, and no additional pain created, as part of MET. The only dangers associated with an approach which calls for direct action of this type is if underlying pathology is ignored. An example of this might be of an acute disc collapse in the spine, causing limitation of movement. In such a case, the pain factor would determine that no real application of MET should be attempted until something had been done about the underlying problem. So, if the factor of increased pain is used as an absolute bar to the use of these methods, then safety is assured. Therefore self-treatment can be safely employed in any restricted joint or muscle if pain is not increased and if it is stopped or varied to a pain-free pattern, or anything more than discomfort is noted.

The various areas of the body will be discussed and illustrated in the text to give guidelines as to general movements and directions of isometric contraction. Suitable methods of applying counterpressure will be outlined.

This will enable most examples of stiffness and restriction to be tackled from this pragmatic viewpoint: "If it's restricted, use MET by taking it to the barrier of movement and then use PIR or RI to release it."

Identification of short, tight muscles

Despite these suggestions it is nevertheless desirable to identify particular muscles which are shortened or which are taut, so that the very best method of using MET can be identified. Once a muscle is identified as being involved in the tightness of a region, specific isometric contractions can be used which will resolve the problem speedily. Thus the examples of tests for tightness given below should be used, where appropriate, to identify specific muscles, or groups of muscles as being culprits and requiring attention.

Tests for tightness

1. Sit on the floor with your legs straight out in front of you. Bend forward with hands outstretched in an attempt to reach your toes. If this is possible, and at the same time your toes can be brought slightly towards your head by flexing your ankle upwards, then there is probably normal length of all

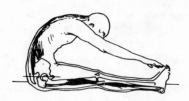

the muscles of the back of your leg, as well as your low back.

2. If you can reach your toes and they tend to point downwards as this is done, then there is probably shortness in the muscles of the back of your lower leg, **gastrocnemius** and **soleus**. These are both postural muscles and should be treated by MET to stretch and relax them. (See individual muscles as listed in chapter 4.)

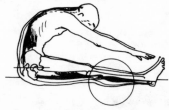

3. If in the same position touching your toes is impossible, even though your lower back is quite rounded and tension is felt strongly in the back of your upper leg, then it is probable that your **hamstrings** are tight. These include **semitendinosus, semimem-**

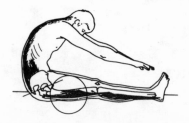

branosus, biceps femoris, and they should be stretched and relaxed by MET.

4. Sometimes the **hamstrings** in only one leg may be shortened. Assess this by sitting as instructed above but with one leg bent, so that the foot of that leg touches the knee of the outstretched leg, and the knee of the bent leg is resting on the floor. Attempt to touch the toes of your outstretched leg, without bending that knee; then change leg positions and attempt to do the same thing with the other leg. Compare the distance which can be reached, as well as the sensation of tightness in the back of each leg and if they are much the same then both hamstrings are probably equally tight, but if there is a noticeable difference then identification of the leg with the major tightness should be simple. Treat this with Muscle Energy methods for the appropriate hamstrings.

5. If, when sitting with both legs outstretched, touching your toes is not possible, and the low back is not well rounded but is more or less upright so that the stretching effort is coming mainly from your upper back, then in all probability your low back muscles are tight and require stretching, using MET.

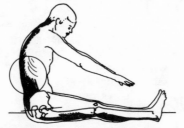

6. If in this same position your low back is actually tilted backwards as the forward bending is attempted, then it may be that both your hamstrings and your low back muscles are tight, and require attention. In such a case there is often a compensatory degree of stretch in the muscles of the upper back and this could do with toning later, after all tightness has been attended to.

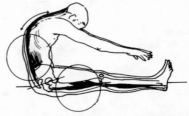

7. Sometimes it is possible to actually reach the toes as a result of excessive stretch in the hamstrings. This stretch is hard to assess without outside observation of the test by an expert, but may be noted as a sensation in which the movement of bend in the back is felt to be coming mainly from the upper back with the lower back felt to be tight, as the bend is performed.

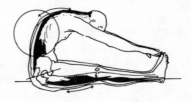

8. If on attempting to touch your toes in this position the furthest that can be reached is roughly knee level or just below, and a sensation of pull is noted in the back of your legs, then probably all the posterior leg muscles (**hamstrings, soleus, gastro-nemius**) are tight as are the low back

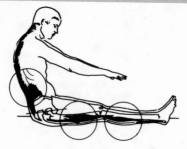

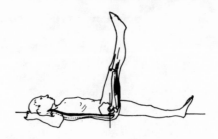

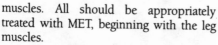

muscles. All should be appropriately treated with MET, beginning with the leg muscles.

9. If, on bending forward, your low back remains in a completely straight or actually backward bent position, then the muscles of your low back are extremely tight and require attention.

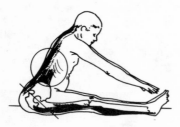

10. Someone is needed to assist in the next test for hamstring and hip flexor status.

Lying on the floor with your back and one leg flat against the floor raise your other leg. This should be able to reach an angle of about 90° (i.e. be able to point straight up at the ceiling) and at the same time your pelvis should be seen to roll slightly backwards to allow this movement to be fully free and your low back should remain constantly in touch with the floor. If, however, your leg cannot be raised beyond about 45°, despite the pelvis rolling some-

what backwards and the spine staying flat on the floor, then your **hamstrings** on that side are short and tight.

11. If in the same position your leg can only be raised to a similar angle (i.e. 45° to 50°) but this time the low back arches upwards as this is achieved, with the pelvis failing to roll backwards, then there is tightness of your low back muscles and of the muscles at the front of the hip of the leg which remained on the floor. These are the flexor muscles of the hips, and guidance will be

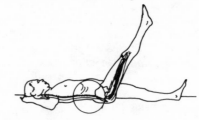

given on using MET to stretch them.

It might be necessary, when doing this test, to actually hold your opposite leg down, as the tested leg is raised.

12. If your leg comes up to about 45°, and your pelvis tilts backwards as it ought to (while the opposite leg is held firm to the table), this indicates that your low back muscles are stretched and that your **hamstrings** are tight.

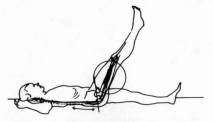

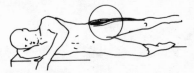

13. If your leg rises to beyond 90°, and your low back stays flat with the pelvic tilt normal (i.e. rolling backwards as the leg is raised) then your **hamstrings** are stretched.

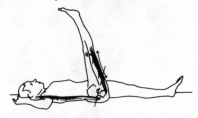

14. If your leg rises to 90°, your pelvis fails to roll backwards and your low back arches, then your hamstrings are stretched whilst your low back muscles and the opposite hip flexors are tight.

15. **The floor is unsuitable for this test since it requires your foot to be able to hang down behind your body. It is possible to self-test for this position, but someone could help in positioning the back leg.**

In a side-lying position on a table your lower leg should be comfortably bent, and your upper leg held backwards of the midline (i.e. slightly extended) so that your foot drops over the edge. The entire trunk of the body should remain in contact with the table when this is being done and should not arch upwards at all. If your foot and leg fail to drop down behind your body, when the pelvis is held in this position, then the **tensor fascia lata** and **iliotibial band** are shortened. This is common in those individuals who have recurrent lower back problems, as these stabilizing, postural soft-tissues frequently shorten and cause imbalance in the pelvic-lumbar mechanics. These musculo-tendinous fibres (**tensor fascia lata**) run down the side of the leg from above the hip to below the knee, and methods of stretching them with MET will be found in the text. (See also Chapter 6.) 16. **Again, a table is needed for the next tests.**

Lying on your back with your buttocks near the end of the table, and one leg flexed with the knee held as close to your chest as possible, the opposite thigh (not the one being flexed) should be parallel with the surface of the table and the lower leg should hang over the edge. If your thigh cannot be held flat in this position, then the hip flexor group of muscles is shortened, which include **iliopsoas**, **rectus femoris** and **tensor fascia lata**. Methods of treating these are described in the text.

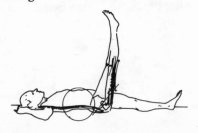

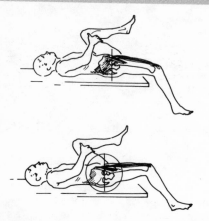

17. If the knee of the leg lying on the table tends to straighten as the thigh is held against the table, and the other knee is pulled to the chest, then rectus femoris is tight. The remaining hip flexors may have allowed hip extension but the shortened

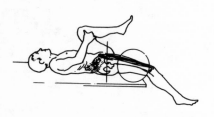

thigh muscle would have transferred the tightness to the knee, making it straighten. 18. Standing with your legs apart about 15 inches, go into a full squat. If it is possible to go right down, with your knees fully bent and your buttocks approaching the floor, without your heels being raised from the floor, then the muscles of the back of your calf are normal. If your heels leave the floor, then the **soleus** muscle is shortened.

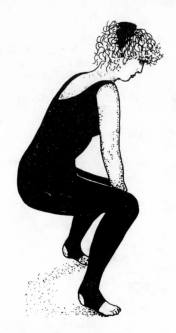

Soleus muscles are shortened since squat position is not achieved with heels flat on floor

19. Lie on your back with legs straight. One ankle is flexed so that the toes come towards the face. This should be a free movement without much resistance until the ankle is well flexed. If there appears to be a limitation to this movement (called dorsiflexion) which disappears when your knee is slightly bent, then **gastrocnemius** is shortened.
20. Sitting on the edge of a table, your hands are placed on the crest of the pelvic bones, fixing the pelvis. Bend, trying to take your forehead to your knees. If this bend fails to reverse the normal curve of your low back, then the **erector spinae** muscles are

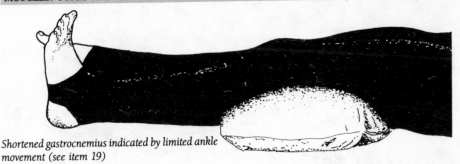

Shortened gastrocnemius indicated by limited ankle movement (see item 19)

shortened. Ideally the bend should be such as to reverse the normal forward curve of the low back.

21. Standing with your legs apart attempt bending as far as possible sideways, running your hand down the side of your thigh. This is done on each side in turn. If, for example, it is not possible to go as far to the left as it is to the right, then the **quadratus lumborum** muscles on the right are probably shortened, thus preventing easy side-bending to the left. If limitation is noted on both sides then both **quadratus lumborum** muscles are short. It should be possible to bend so that your hands reach to between mid-calf and the ankles. **Ensure that no**

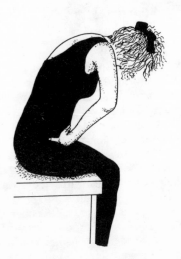

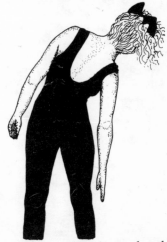

Lumbar curve is reversed which shows normal erector spinae muscles (see item 20)

Side bend shows relative tightness of quadratus lumborum when compared with other side (see item 21)

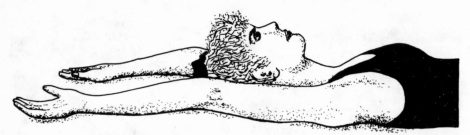

Test successfully completed as entire length of arm touches surface (see item 22)

forwards bending is combined with side-bending in this test. MET for such shortening is described in the text.

22. Lying on the floor or table stretch your arms over the top of your head. Keep your back flat all the time and flex your knees and hips. The entire length of your arm should be able to be rested flat on the floor or table, above your head. If this is not possible, then tightness exists in the adductors and internal rotators of the arms, including **pectoralis major** and **minor**, **latissiumus dorsi**, **teres major**, **subscapularis** and **the rhomboids**.

23. Sitting at a table turn your head as far

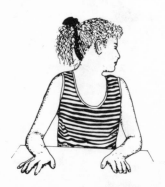

one way as possible and then assess its range by doing the same on the other side. If it is possible to go further in one direction than the other, then there is shortening of muscles on the side opposite to the way in which you are looking, (i.e. if the head turns further to the right than the left then there is muscle shortening on the right). This could involve a number of muscles with fibres at the side of the neck, including **sterno-cleido mastoid**, **scaleni**, **posterior cervical** and upper branches of **trapezius**. MET measures for the neck will help in general freeing of the area.

Next drop your head forward into full flexion. (Your chin should be able to touch your chest.) Shortness in the **semispinalis**, **longissimus**, the upper branches of **trapezius** and other small muscles lying at the back of the neck, could be the cause of any restriction preventing this.

24. Tilt your head into a position as far back as possible, so that you are looking up at the ceiling. If this is difficult then there could be shortening in the **scaleni**, **sternomastoid**, **longus capitus** and/or **longus coli** muscles which lie at the front and side of the neck. Sitting as above, lay your head as close as possible to your shoulder on one side and then the other, comparing for freedom of movement. The side which is shortened is

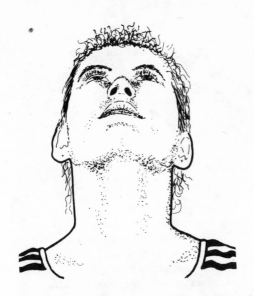
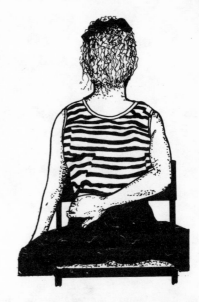

the one opposite the side where limitation is noted (i.e. If it is more difficult to take the head sideways to the right then there is shortening of the lateral muscles in the neck on the left.) This probably involves the upper fibres of the **trapezius** and **sterno mastoid** on that side. A simple test to assess whether the **sternomastoid muscles** are short is to lie on your back, without a pillow and to then slowly lift your head as though you were trying to touch your chin to your upper chest. If, as you start this lift, the chin pokes forwards, rather than the forehead rising first with the chin staying 'tucked in', then **sternomastoid** is definitely shortened. You may need someone to watch you do this to make this judgement.

25. Rotation of your lower arm may be compared by extending the arms one at a time and turning the clenched fist, first as far one way as possible, and then the other. Compare the ranges of movement in the two arms in the various directions. Limitation might involve **infraspinatus**, **deltoid**, **subscapularis** and others. In this case, MET is easily applied to these regions in self-treatment and the text will explain this.

26. Test your **biceps** muscle by sitting and reaching with one hand at a time behind the back and trying to reach the opposite hip. If there is limitation on one side the difference will be noted. MET stretching of the **biceps** is described in the text.

27. Lying on your back, assess which of your lower legs is turned out more than the other. (They may both be turned out.) If one is noticeably so, and there is a history of low back or leg pain on that side, then the **piriformis** muscle on that side may be shortened. MET treatment for this is simple

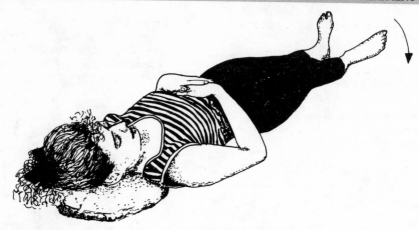

and is described in the text.

28. Lying on your back with legs flat on the floor put first one and then the other leg out sideways as far as possible, and compare the range. If one is more limited than the other then the adductors of the leg on that side are shortened, and may be treated with MET. If both are shortened then only a limited excursion sideways will be possible. (It should be possible to carry the leg outwards a good 45° from the midline.)

Having taken your leg away from the midline, knee kept straight, allow the knee to bend, and note whether your leg can now travel further outwards than previously. If it cannot and there appears to be some limitation of the range of movement in comparison with the other leg, the MET treatment method should be applied with your knee bent, and with your leg out as in the test. If, however, there appears to be limitation but your leg does travel outwards

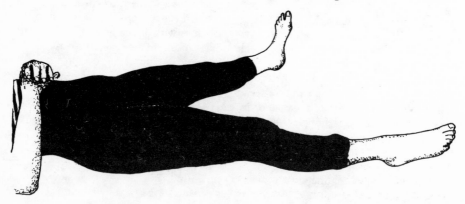

further when your knee is bent, treat with the leg straight.

29. Testing the tightness in individual fingers and toes as well as wrists and ankles, is largely a matter of comparison with the normal, and of contrasting the two sides of the body. Use the guidelines of taking any restricted joint to its pain-free limit in the direction of the restriction, and then use PIR and RI to release tightness in the muscles, by using either the tight muscles or their antagonists to go towards or away from the barrier, with counterpressure preventing movement.

30. By opening your mouth widely it is possible to observe whether there is a deviation to one side. If the jaw deviates to the left as it opens then there is a restriction or shortening in the muscles on the left side, for example in the **masseter** or **temporalis**, and appropriate MET methods are given in the text to normalize these. **The tempero-mandibular joint may be at fault, however, and this can call for expert manipulative attention, especially if there is accom-**

mainly sideways as the breath is taken in, then this is normal. If, however, there is a movement upwards of the hands (or your shoulders) at this time then inappropriate muscles are being used in the breathing action, and attention should be paid to these. Often noted in such cases is shortness in the **levator scapulae**, **pectoralis** (upper fibres), **trapezius**, **scaleni** and other muscles of the neck and upper chest which should not be primarily involved in the breathing action. MET measures directed towards these as well as restraining in correct breathing patterns is necessary.

32. Rest the fingers of one hand on the outer end of the collar bone of the other side. Raise your arm of that other side upwards so that it is rising partly sideways and partly forwards (about 45° forwards). As your arm passes the horizontal and begins to go upwards, your fingers resting on the very

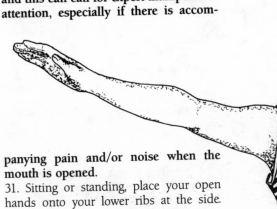

panying pain and/or noise when the mouth is opened.

31. Sitting or standing, place your open hands onto your lower ribs at the side. Breathe in deeply and note the movement of your hands. If they appear to be moving

end of the collar bone should feel this sink a little, and this happens to allow the joint in your shoulder to move freely as your arm rises further. Your collar bone may however be felt to rise instead of fall, and this indicates dysfunction at the acromioclavicular joint, involving possibly any or all of the following: **levator scapulae, deltoid, teres major** and **minor, supraspinatus** and **infraspinatus**, and the **serratus anterior** muscles. Methods for releasing the muscles of the shoulder using MET will be given in the text.

Tests for muscle weakness

It is not proposed to individually describe the testing of weakness in the muscles of the body, since few of these can be adequately self-tested and accurate assessment requires someone to be able to grade the results. There is never, or almost never, an 'all or nothing' response in terms of strength or weakness in muscles. By this it is meant that few muscles are so weak as to be totally unable to respond, unless paralysis is involved. Therefore, weakness might be slight or of medium, moderate or great degree. Comparison with other muscles as well as knowledge whereby comparison can be made with norms in the population in general, taking into account age, sex, body-type, occupation and other factors, is necessary.

In the context of self-help measures, weakness of muscles which is obvious, and for which there is no reason, should lead to enquiries being made from an expert. If the reasons are known, (prolonged disuse as in

an immobilized limb after an injury, for example), then this may be helped by use of the isotonic or isokinetic measures discussed previously.

The major aim of the description of MET methods in this book is the introduction of safe measures whereby tight, shortened muscles may be released and relaxed. In describing MET methods, isotonic methods of strengthening weak muscles have been mentioned, and these are safe and available wherever weak muscles are noted.

However, the emphasis must be on releasing tight muscles, as these are often the primary reason for weakness in their antagonists. The antagonists' condition improves spontaneously when the shortened, taut muscles are freed.

Whilst exercise and toning of weak muscles may be attempted by various other means than MET, releasing tight muscles in a self-help context is a contribution unique to MET, which recognizes that attention to tight muscles should be the primary aim in any attempt at restoration of good body mechanics.

If there are known muscle weaknesses, treatment of these should be left until tight, shortened muscles have been successfully dealt with, at which time weak muscles should be given attention if they have not fully recovered tone and strength spontaneously.

In this connection, the methods associated with Applied Kinesiology (AK) should be mentioned. This American system maintains that tight muscles are the result of weak muscles which require strengthening by a variety of means incorporated into AK. However, all the evidence of major researchers into muscle physiology and body mechanics indicates the precise opposite.

Vladimir Janda, a renowned physiologist, states the case thus in *The Neurobiological Mechanisms in Manipulative Therapy* (Plenum Press, 1980) when he says:

> In pathogenesis as well as in treatment of muscle imbalance and back problems, tight muscles play a more important and perhaps even primary role in comparison to weak muscles.
>
> Clinical experience and therapeutic results support the assumption that tight muscles act in an inhibitory way on antagonists therefore it does not seem reasonable to start with strengthening of the weakened muscles as most exercise programmes do.
>
> It has been clinically proved that it is better to stretch the tight muscles first, thus inhibiting the weakened, inhibited antagonists.
>
> It is not exceptional that, after stretching of the tight muscle, the strength of the inhibited weakened antagonist improves spontaneously, sometimes immediately, sometimes

within a few days, without any additional treatment.

Other experts in the field such as Karel Lewit MD, author of the book *Manipulative Therapy in Rehabilitation of the Locomotor System* (Butterworths, 1985) makes this a firm injunction:

> First the hyperactive muscles showing increased tension (spasm, trigger points, shortening) should be relaxed; *after* this, the weak (inhibited, flabby) muscles should be trained. This order is mandatory, in particular if the muscles with increased tension are the antagonists of the weak muscles.

Here then, is a plan of action:

- Identify tight, shortened muscles.
- Use MET to relax and release these.
- Then, if there remains any noticeable weakness, employ exercise or isotonic MET methods to strengthen these.

The AK injunction to strengthen weak muscles first is based upon an inaccurate reading of the physiology of the body.

Important Caution

There are times when symptoms of extreme tightness in muscles should be left alone.

If there exists in the bones of the spine, for example, a condition of osteoporosis, (a decalcification or 'thinning' of the bones), then there is frequently an accompanying contraction or spasm of the overlying muscles. If a vertebrae actually collapses in such a situation, there is great pain and

extreme spasm in the muscle of the area. This is protective, and designed by the body to prevent movement which could produce pain, or worse, an actual fracture of the bone.

Similarly, if there were a tumour in a bone in the lower spine, or neck, for example, then this could be accompanied by a similar protective spasm, for similar reasons.

In neither of these examples would

MET be of any use since any relaxation it achieved, (and this would be unlikely under these conditions anyway), would obviously be against the best interests of the body, which requires, and should receive, immobilization of the damaged area.

In a joint which is actively inflamed and swollen due, for example, to rheumatoid arthritis, there is little that MET could do for the tissues of the area which would be of value. In such conditions, the tense and/or weak muscles can often be helped by MET and other methods, once the inflammation is reduced somewhat, but in the very acute phases these tissues do not require activity, however gentle. Arthritic and other damaged joints can be helped by MET to regain some freedom of movement, but not if the methods produce pain, which should in any condition be seen as indicating that MET, or any other self-help method, should be stopped. Furthermore, not all symptoms need to be overcome. Many symptoms such as pain and restricted movement, need to be recognized for what they are, as in the examples given above, in which they show an intelligent protective role for pain or tight muscles.

It is always important to try to find out why there is pain or stiffness before trying to change behaviour of muscles since, whilst most stiff muscles and joints can be helped by MET, caution should be exercised in situations such as those described above. In any condition of pain, stiffness, or disability which does not resolve itself fairly rapidly, it is suggested that a qualified osteopathic or chiropractic practitioner should be consulted.

The methods described in this book are used by many such practitioners, along with a host of other specialized methods which can comprehensively assist in the normalization of musculoskeletal problems, where possible.

In dealing with the pains and dysfunctions of the body the osteopath does not look at the local symptoms and area alone, but at its relationship with the other parts of the body as well as at the relationship of the body as a whole with its environment. Such questions might include:

- How is the body used and abused in daily life?
- What inborn defects exist and what has resulted from the vicissitudes and traumas of life?
- How do posture, reflex activity, occupation, emotional stress, sporting activity etc. relate to the current situation?

These are all vital questions which often require answers before a condition of bodily dysfunction can be normalized.

Treatment of symptoms alone is never enough. The self-help methods, as adapted in this book, should not replace expert advice, but should be used as first-aid and as a source of guidance for ongoing maintenance of mobility, once this has been regained.

4

Muscle Energy Techniques in action — treatment and self-treatment methods

Active Home treatment methods for normalizing muscular imbalance in back conditions

Statistics show that most backaches are better within 3 weeks whether the treatment received involves active manipulation, traction, physiotherapy or total rest (an approach which carries with it economic and practical difficulties). Only a small percentage of back problems last for as long as six weeks or require specialized attention. *None of the methods listed above ensure that relapse will not occur.*

Experts such as Doctors Karel Lewit and Vladimir Janda in Czechoslovakia and H. Schmid (of the Department of Physical Medicine, Lindenhof Hospital, Bern, Switzerland) have developed a series of exercises which focus on stretching tight postural muscles (see chapters 1 and 2) followed by toning weak phasic muscles. They claim that this approach does indeed help ensure the avoidance of relapse of many low back problems. The stretching exercises appropriate to the individual patient's needs (hamstrings, psoas, tensor facia lata, adductors, soleus, gastrocnemius, piriformis, quadratus, spinal erectors, abdominals, pectoralis major, trapezius, sternomastoid, levator scapulae etc) are done for five minutes several times daily. These are integrated into a daily routine once recovery is established to maintain mobility and keep problems at bay.

Unless you are lucky enough to have access to the expert guidance of these fine doctors, or of specialists in spinal mechanics such as osteopathic or chiropractic practitioners, identification of which muscles need stretching in any particular case can be best achieved by following the self-testing procedures for tight muscle groups as outlined in chapter 3. Methods for normalizing those in need of stretching are detailed in this chapter.

Muscles involved:

Sternomastoid, scalene, posterior cervicals, upper branches of trapezius, semispinalis, longissimus, longus capitus, longus coli and other smaller muscles of the neck.
These support and move the head and neck in various directions.

Associated problems:

Headache, neck stiffness and pain. These muscles should be searched for trigger points which are often involved in referred pain and other symptoms related to the head, eyes and face. (See Chapter 5.)

Position and method

After each of the following 6 isometric exercises you should either take your head/neck as far as is comfortable (that is, stretch it gently) in the direction towards which it was being isometrically pushed *or* in the opposite direction to that push, in order to gain an increased range of motion where stiffness was previously felt. In this way you will take advantage of both post isometric relaxation (PIR) or reciprocal inhibition (RI) as described in chapters 1 and 2. Unlike the methods listed later in this chapter, for specific muscles, these 6 exercises are aimed at general mobility improvement.

1. Sit at a table with your elbows resting on it, and your hands at the sides of your head. Stabilizing your head with your open hands, try first to tilt your head sideways against your right hand, using only about a quarter of the available strength in your muscles. As you do this, breathe in and hold your breath for the duration of the contraction, which should last for 5-7 seconds. Relax the effort as you release your breath. Repeat this in the same direction two or three times for the same length of time and using the same degree of effort.

  Perform the same isometric contraction, but this time pushing to the left, for the same length of time. Repeat this two or three times.

2. Place your hands together over your forehead with your neck flexed and your head resting on your hands. Push your hands against your forehead and your forehead against your hands in an isometric contraction which begins with a deep breath, held for the duration of the contraction, i.e. about 7 seconds. Ease the pressure slowly as you release your breath. Repeat this several times.

3. With your neck flexed, and your chin near your chest, place one (or both) hand(s)

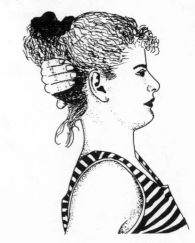

See item 4 on page 56

on the back of your head and begin a contraction in which your head is being pushed backwards as your hand(s) restrain it. Breathe in at the beginning and hold for 5-7 seconds. Breathe out and release pressure slowly.

Repeat the contraction two or three times.

4. Carefully move your head backwards to look upwards at the ceiling. Restraining your head by pressure on your forehead, gently attempt to push your head upright again. Use only about 10 per cent of strength in this position, which can be uncomfortable if greater effort is used.

Repeat several times holding your breath with each contraction.

5. Sitting upright, pull your chin backwards as though it were going through the back of your neck. This opens the facets of the spine in the region. In this position, place a hand on your chin and restrain effort to return it to its normal, jutting position, breathing in at the start and holding for 5-7 seconds, before releasing and repeating.

6. Place your left hand on your left cheek, and with this restrain a turning of your head to the left. Again combine breathing and contraction for 5-7 seconds, before releasing and repeating. Do the same on the right side.

The sequence of directions of movement described is not important, but if there is any specific direction in which limitation is noted, then take the head as far as you can in that direction before restraining the head at that point, and either try to take it further towards that barrier or away from the barrier, resisting isometrically. The timing

and breathing should be the same as above.

Repetition should be begun at the furthest, pain-free, limit in the restricted direction.

The use of general neck techniques such as these is appropriate for most forms of headache and where the neck is commonly stiff, especially if this follows being in a static position such as typing, driving etc. for a long period.

If before commencing the series of isometric neck releasing exercises described above there was a feeling of general stiffness or restriction, this should be much relieved afterwards.

A specific indicator exists when there is shortening of the muscles at the back of the neck which would be stretched by use of

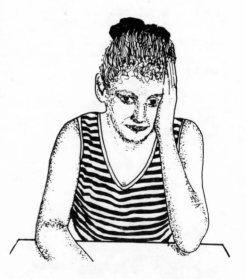

Isometric contraction of muscles on left side of neck

exercises 3 and 5 above (see also pages 58 and 59).

In this sequence, most of the major and minor neck muscles will be released.

Sitting upright, take the chin as close as comfortably is possible towards the upper border of the breastbone (sternum).

If shortened, these muscles will prevent the chin from coming almost to a point of being able to touch this region.

If three or more finger widths' distance separate chin from breastbone, then these post-cervical muscles are very short, and almost certainly contain trigger points.

Assess this distance again after the iso-metric manuoeuvres, outlined above.

Specific neck-muscle releasing methods will be found in this section as we progress through individual muscle problems. However, the general measures described will often be all that is required to keep the neck supple.

Both PIR and RI will have been used in the methods described, and these can also be used in treating someone else, in which case the counterpressure would be applied for them by the operator's hands.

Note: **Remember to stretch painlessly the muscles used, or their antagonists, after each isometric contraction.**

Muscles involved:	Short extensors of the neck. These muscles are the small ones at the base of the skull and they have control of fine movement. They are subject to shortening.
Associated problems:	Neck stiffness and head or eye problems.

Position and method

Sit on a low chair leaning backwards. Place your fingers on the base of your skull (where the skull meets the neck) whilst the thumbs are on the cheek bones, just below the eyes. Draw your chin back into your neck (double chin position) and in this position, stabilizing the whole area with your hands, breathe in and look upwards at the same time (eyes only, no conscious neck movement). There will be a tendency at this moment to raise your head *which your hands should restrain*. This eye position is held (with the breath) for five seconds, and then as the breath is slowly released, take your chin a little closer to your throat, thus

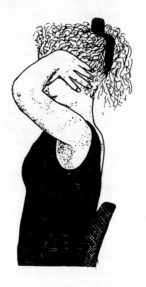

stretching the muscles of the upper neck. (This technique is enhanced by simultaneously casting your eyes downward.) Repeat. Leaning backwards onto the chair will bring your chin closer to your throat on relaxation.

This MET method illustrates the use of breathing and eye movement to introduce muscular contraction, which is isometrically resisted by hand counterpressure. The degree of muscular effort is not great, but the relaxation which can be achieved by several repetitions of this exercise makes it a powerful aid in normalizing tension at the base of the skull, a common factor in headache and eyestrain conditions.

Left *isometric contraction of short extensor muscles of neck resisted by hand contact*

Muscle involved:	Levator scapulae. This emerges from the spinous processes of the top four vertebrae of the spine and inserts into the top of the shoulder blade. Its function relates to shoulder stability and arm movement.
Associated problems:	Pain in the upper neck (side) and upper aspect of shoulder blade. Trigger points in this muscle cause pain in the neck, shoulder and shoulder blade. The muscle may be extra tense if you suffer from asthma.

Position and method

1. Lie on a bed or on the floor with a pillow under your head. Reach down as far as is comfortable with your hand on the affected side and place the palm side of your hand under your buttock or upper thigh, holding it there. Your shoulder on this side should

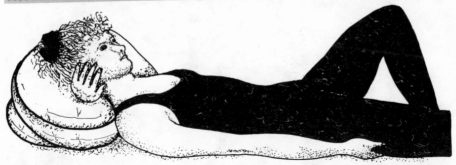

Isometric contraction of right levator scapulae muscle

be pulled down by this action as far as is comfortable.

2. Your other hand should reach up behind your head so that your fingers rest over your ear on the opposite side. This hand should pull your head sideways, with slight rotation, towards the side opposite the affected muscle. All the slack should be taken up so that with the one arm pulling downwards and the neck and head being pulled to the opposite side, a good deal of tension is being exerted on the muscles of the region.

3. You should now turn only your eyes (not your head) to the affected side at the same time as taking and holding a deep breath. There will be an automatic tendency to

want to turn your head in the direction in which your eyes are looking. This must be resisted or it will release the tension in the muscles necessary to produce the contractile force to create the isometric contraction which is acting against the counterpressure of your hand on your head.

4. After 5-7 seconds, breathe out. At the same time, turn your eyes towards the opposite side, away from the affected side. As you breathe out pull your head a little further away from the affected side, taking it to its new barrier of resistance, and increasing the tension in the shortened muscle.

5. Repeat the procedure several times always incorporating the eye movement, the deep breath and the steady pull with the hand on the head.

Muscle involved:	Trapezius (upper fibres). The trapezius is a flat, triangular muscle covering the back of the neck and shoulders. Its fibres run from the base of the skull to the outer aspect of the

collar bone, and it draws the head backwards and stabilizes and lifts the shoulder when arm movement is taking place.

Associated problems:

Neck and shoulder and arm problems. Trigger points in this muscle can cause pain in the jaw region and the side of the head, and may cause problems in the ears and eyes. (Conjunctivitis etc.)

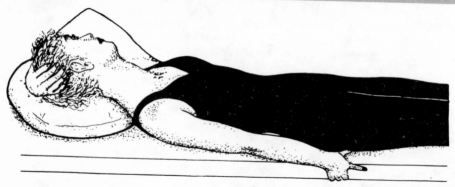

Isometric contraction of upper fibres of right trapezius muscle

Position and method

1. Lie on your back on a bed or table. Grip the edge of the bed or table with the hand on your affected side with your arm at about a 45° angle from your shoulder, pointing downwards. With your other hand, reach across the top of your head and pull your head as far to the side opposite the affected muscle as is comfortably possible.
2. At the point where all the slack has been taken out, turn your eyes only to the affected side and breathe in deeply. This will tend to place strain on your tense muscles, since the eye movement will automatically produce a contraction in the muscles of that side as your head prepares to turn. This tendency to turn should be resisted by the hand on your head, and this provides the counterpressure. After a count of 5-7 seconds release your breath, and at the same time turn your eyes to the side to which your head is being pulled by your hand. This pull is maintained all the time, and with the relaxation which accompanies exhalation the pull is increased slightly to take out more slack in the muscles.

3. The breathing in and the eye movement to the affected side should then be repeated several times more, combined with relaxation and stretching towards the new barrier, as above.

This same position is used when supplying the counterpressure for someone else, i.e. one hand on the shoulder and the other on the side of the head, applying stretch to the tissues as resistance is applied during contractions. Eye movement and breathing are as above.

It is permissible to introduce a slight muscular effort as well as the eye movement if no pain is noted as the range of motion increases after each contraction. In such a case, as well as the eye movement a small degree of effort could be introduced, in which an attempt could be made to take the restrained head towards the fixed shoulder and also to shrug that shoulder partially towards the ear. The hand holding the side of the table prevents this shoulder from moving, and the isometric contraction induced should result in increased range of motion of the head, towards the opposite shoulder, afterwards.

Muscle involved:	Sternocleidomastoid. (Usually called sternomastoid.) This runs from the top of the breast bone and inserts into the mastoid bone behind the ear. Its function is as a neck stabilizer and neck flexor as well as lifting some of the structures of the chest in breathing.
Associated problems:	Pain on the outer end of the collar bone; pain in the upper neck. Trigger points in the muscle produce pain in the region of the jaw, throat and forehead. Active triggers have been associated with sinus problems, allergies and alterations in skin function on the face and head (greasy or very dry).

Position and method

1. Lie on your back on a table so that your head is turned away from the affected side, with the top of your head over the edge of the table and the base of your skull resting

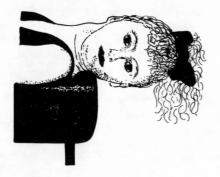

Above *isometric contraction of right sternomastoid muscle*

Below *relaxation and stretch of right sternomastoid muscle after isometric contraction — using gravity as counterweight*

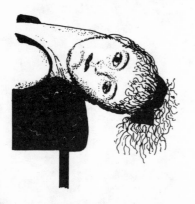

on the edge. In this position gravity will be exerting a pull on the muscle as your head hangs slightly down.

2. With your head turned as far as is com-fortable and hanging slightly as indicated, your eyes should be turned towards the ceiling as a deep breath is taken. As this is done the muscle will contract slightly.

3. The breath and eye position are held for 5–7 seconds at which point the breath should be released and your eyes turned in the direction in which your head is held. At this stage your head should be allowed to sink a little further towards the floor, for up to half a minute.

4. Take another deep breath and turn your eyes to the ceiling to again contract the muscle against the counterforce of gravity.

It is essential that between such efforts, as the breath is released, a complete relaxation is allowed so that maximum stretch is placed on the muscle. The sequence should be repeated three or four times.

If you have experienced pain with gentle pressure exerted on the top vertebrae of your spine, then this self-treatment will often relieve the condition. As in the previous example, it may be desirable to introduce a slight additional muscular effort.

If so, then as you breathe in, and your eyes turn to the ceiling, a slight lift of your head should be introduced, raising it no more than a centimetre or two.

This position should be held for the duration of the breath/eye position and released coincidentally, i.e. after 5–7 seconds, allowing the subsequent gravity-induced stretch to continue for 30 seconds or so.

Muscle involved:

Scalene.
This muscle has three divisions:
  Anticus which runs from the front of
  the lateral processes of the 3rd to the
  6th cervical (neck) vertebrae to the
  1st rib.
  Medius which runs from the lateral
  (transverse) processes of the 2nd to
  the 7th cervical vertebrae to the 1st
  (and sometimes the 2nd) rib(s).
  Posterior which runs from the
  transverse processes of the 5th to 7th
  cervical vertebrae to the 2nd rib.

Associated problems:

These usually include faulty respiration,
especially feelings of being unable to
take a deep breath. They may contain
trigger points which refer pain to the
head and face.

Position and method

1. Lie on your back with your head a little
over the head of the bed or table so that it
hangs slightly down. Your head should be
turned away from the side of your scalene
to be treated. If your head is thus hanging
down in a backwards bent and rotated
position to the left, there would be tension
on the right scalene muscles. Depending
upon the degree of rotation of your head
this would involve scalenus anticus,
medius or posterior.

The more rotation that is introduced, the
more likely there is to be involvement of
posterior or medius divisions. If the muscle
has been gently palpated to see where
tenderness or fibrous changes (or trigger

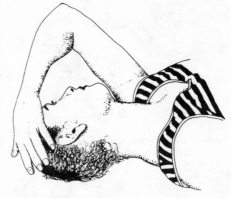

points) are present, it will be possible to
note, when the self-treatment is performed,
whether or not these fibres are contracting.
2. With your head thus turned to the left,

place your left hand on the right side of your forehead/face and use this to resist the contraction which occurs when a deep breath is taken in. Your eyes should be turned as far as possible to the right. At the same time, a slight lift of your head is made, together with a slight turn towards the right. No movement should be allowed because of your restraining hand on the head.

The amount of lift and turn used should be minimal. Hold this for 7–10 seconds and then, as your breath is released and your eyes turn all the way to the left, allow your muscles to stretch, via gravity's pull on the head, for about ten seconds. Repeat the exercise.

To involve different fibres of the muscle turn your head more or less to the side. After several repetitions re-test the muscle for tenderness and for the presence of trigger points.

Muscle involved:

Pectoralis major.
This is a fan-shaped muscle which runs from the inner half of the collar bone inserting into the upper arm. It helps to raise the arm at the shoulder and is often contracted when arm pain is noted.

Associated problems:

Round-shouldered posture.
Trigger points in this muscle produce pain in the upper chest muscles usually to the side of the nipple and running towards the armpit. This muscle is often tense in stress conditions.

Isometric contraction of pectoralis major

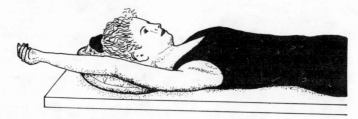

Position and method

1. Lying on your back on a table or bed with your affected side close to the edge. Your arm should be outstretched to your side and hanging palm upwards. The edge of the bed should be supporting your upper arm

Relaxation and stretch of pectoralis major after isometric contraction

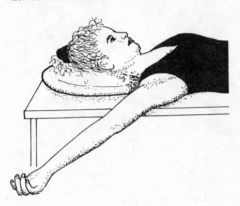

a few inches below your shoulder joint.

2. Having achieved a maximum degree of stretch in this manner, take a deep breath and at the same time raise your extended arm about an inch. Hold this position for the duration of the held breath, which should be about 7-10 seconds. Gravity is acting as the counterforce in this manoeuvre.

3. As you release your breath, gently stretch your arm further. This should be done very slowly so as not to irritate the muscle. Repeat a deep breath with a slight raising of the arm towards the ceiling and hold for the duration of the normal isometric contraction. Again breathe out and slowly allow your arm to fully stretch towards the floor, putting stretch on the affected muscle. Repeat three or four times. Holding a light weight in the hand (for example, a can of vegetables) can assist as this increases the gravity induced stretch after the contraction.

Assisted isometric contraction of pectoralis major

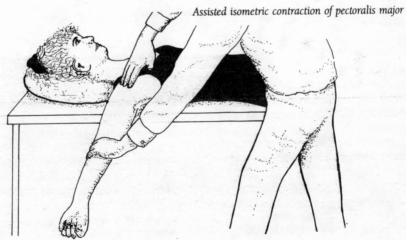

In treating someone else, the counter-pressure is supplied by the hand which holds the upper arm as it attempts to rise.

Not much effort should be used, as the breath is taken in. In all other ways the method is identical to self-treatment.

Muscle involved:

Supraspinatus.
This runs from the ridge on your shoulder blade outwards to your upper arm, which it assists in sideways movements.

Associated problems:

Difficulty raising arm sideways.
Triggers in this muscle refer pain to an area between the neck and shoulder, mainly on the outer aspect of the shoulder joint itself and running down the outer arm. 'Frozen shoulder' conditions usually involve this muscle.

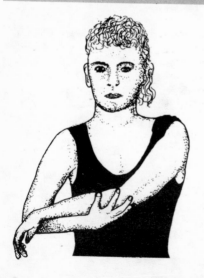

Position and method

1. Sitting. The arm on your affected side should be bent at the elbow and carried across your chest so that your elbow is as far across as is comfortable. Your other hand should grasp your elbow and cup it to exert a pull towards the opposite shoulder, increasing stretch of the affected muscle. As a deep breath is taken, your elbow should be pushed slightly back towards your affected side, against the resistance of your hand holding it. Hold this for about 10 seconds.

Left *isometric contraction of left supraspinatus muscle — self treatment*

The pressure should be moderate and not by any means full strength. On breathing out, release the contraction gently, not suddenly, and take your arm a little further towards the opposite side by drawing it across your chest.

2. When maximum painless stretch has been reached, the breath and isometric contraction should be performed again for a further 10 seconds. Repeat the sequence three or four times or until no more gain is noted in terms of your arm being able to travel further.

Treatment by someone else involves them standing behind and holding the arm (in the position described above) which is prevented from being taken sideways (into abduction) during the breathing-in phase of the cycle. Minimal effort is required for good results.

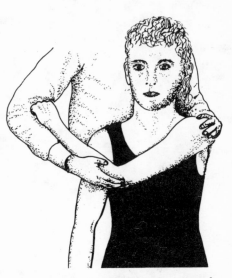

Isometric contraction of left supraspinatus muscle — assisted

Muscle involved:	Infraspinatus. This thick, triangular muscle runs from the inner border of your shoulder blade to the back of your upper arm which it stabilizes and assists in outward rotation and lifting.
Associated problems:	Problems relate to the functions of the arm with which the muscle is connected, which are raising and rotation. Trying to turn the arm outwards against resistance would be painful if the muscle was disturbed. Trigger points found in it refer pain to the outer upper arm, especially to the

front of the shoulder, and down the arm as far as the two fingers next to the thumb. The muscle may be involved in 'frozen shoulder' conditions.

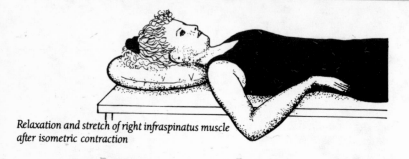

Relaxation and stretch of right infraspinatus muscle after isometric contraction

Position and method

1. Lie on a bed with your affected arm over the side. Your upper arm should extend sideways from your shoulder and your elbow should be bent so that it forms a right angle, with your lower arm directed towards the foot of the bed. Your arm should be pos-

itioned so that your palm faces the floor. Your upper arm should be resting on the edge of the bed.
2. In this position allow your arm to relax fully, placing maximum stretch on the muscle via the pull of gravity on your lower

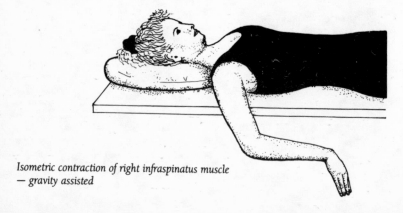

Isometric contraction of right infraspinatus muscle — gravity assisted

arm. At this point raise your forearm towards the ceiling by no more than an inch or two. Hold this for 15-20 seconds before slowly releasing and allowing the muscle to be taken again to its maximum degree of pain-free stretch. Hold this for an equal length of time.

3. Repeat the raising of your forearm by an inch or so as described. This provides contraction of the muscle against gravity's counterpressure. Relaxation also employs gravity's pull to stretch the muscle fully. Repeat three or four times, at any one self-treatment session.

Muscle involved:

Subscapularis.
This runs from the outer two-thirds of the surface of the front of your shoulder blade into your upper arm which it helps to raise and rotate.

Associated problems:

Since this muscle assists in raising your arm and turning it inwards, shortening results in limitations of these movements, and is often associated with 'frozen shoulder'. Trigger points found in this muscle send pain into the arm, across the shoulder blade, mainly to the back of the shoulder joint.

Position and method

Lie on your back with your upper arm extended sideways from your shoulder, over the edge of the table, and with your elbow bent at right angles, so that your upper arm is palm upwards with your hand at a level with, or above, your head. However, the condition of your shoulder may limit your ability to reach this position and so the maximum possible, pain-free stretch into this position should be attempted. With your arm thus positioned, your upper arm is allowed to stretch as much as possible, at which time your wrist and forearm should be raised an inch or so and held for about 15-20 seconds, as your breath is held. During the release of both your breath and the lift, which should be slow, your arm should be allowed to fall gently as far as it can, introducing maximum stretch to the muscle. Holding a light weight (e.g. a can of vegetables) in the hand can assist as this increases the gravity induced stretch after the contraction.

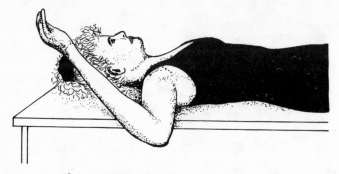

Above *isometric contraction of right subscapularis muscle — gravity assisted*

Below *relaxation and stretch of right subscapularis after isometric contraction*

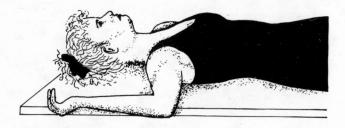

This stretch is held for the same length of time as the contraction, which should be repeated, as above, three or four times, or until maximum release has been achieved.

The exercise is particularly effective in helping restore motion to a 'frozen shoulder'.

Muscles involved:

Upper Erector spinae.
These are the postural muscles which extend from the base of your spine to your neck and which provide stability and some limited movement.

Associated problems:

The supporting muscles of your upper spine which also stabilize your head and which are involved in bending the head backwards and tilting the head upwards are often shortened and in need of relaxation, especially in relation to headaches and stiff neck. Triggers in this area can refer pain to the head, neck and shoulder blade. Turning the neck and looking up and down might be limited.

Position and method

1. Lie face downwards on a bed or table, with the upper part of your head and face over the edge so that, when your head is turned, there is support at a point between your ear and chin. Thus, only that part of your head from about your mouth upwards is over the edge. Turn your head towards the side of the shortened muscles.

2. For MET affecting the upper fibres, you should fully relax your head in this position, and then, on breathing in, lift it slightly (i.e. your whole head should be raised sideways towards the ceiling), by half an inch. Gravity is producing the counterpressure and this contraction should be held for 5-7 seconds. As you release your breath your head should be relaxed to encourage a stretching of the shortened muscles. Repeat this sequence several times.

If the fibres of your lower neck and upper thoracic spine are to be treated, then the raising of your head should be greater, perhaps an inch or more, or until the

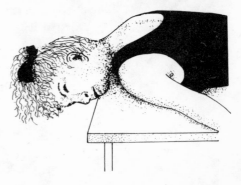

Isometric contraction of erector spinae muscles on the left of the neck and upper back — after the contraction the muscles are relaxed to allow the head to hang further thereby placing stretch on the fibres on the left side

muscles of your lower neck are felt to be contracting. All other aspects of the method are the same.

Treatment by someone else involves the subject being seated, with the helper standing behind and to the side, with one hand fixing the shoulder of the side to be treated, whilst the other hand encircles the head and pulls it gently into rotation, forward bending and sidebending, away from the affected side.

Isometric contraction is brought about by the subject breathing deeply and looking to the affected side, while the helper resists any slight movement brought about by the resulting contraction.

Timing etc. is as above.

If it is thought necessary to increase the degree of isometric contraction because of insufficient release by the method described above, the subject (patient) should employ a slight muscular effort as the breath is taken in and the eyes turn. This effort should, of course, be minimal.

Muscles involved:	Mid-spine Erector Spinae. Postural muscles associated with the vertebrae.
Associated problems:	Stiffness and pain in the back. Triggers from this muscle group can affect the back, ribs and shoulders.

Position and method

1. Sitting. The hand on the side of the back NOT being treated should be placed on the top of your head. Twist your trunk away from the side of the affected muscles and pull your head into a position of rotation, bending sideways and forwards, also away from the affected side. The hand on the affected side should reach across the opposite thigh to rest in a position which maximizes the degree of rotation desired. It is possible to localize the effective contraction by bending and rotating in this way until stretch is felt in the appropriate area of your back.

2. Having established this position, turn your eyes towards the affected side. At the same time, a deep breath is taken in. This produces a tendency for the affected muscles to contract, which is resisted by the pull from the hand on your head. As you release the breath, after 5-10 seconds, your eyes should turn towards the side towards which rotation is directed, (i.e. away from the affected side) and a degree of additional stretch will then be available. Any additional looseness should then be taken out by the forwards pull of the hand on your head and additional rotation. Repeat the measure as above, two or three times more, or until maximum rotation has been achieved.

If this is assisted by someone else, the hands of the person being treated may be interlocked at the back of the head. If the

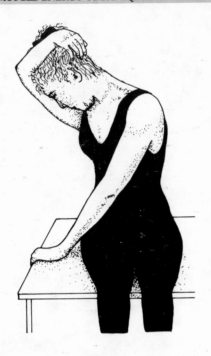

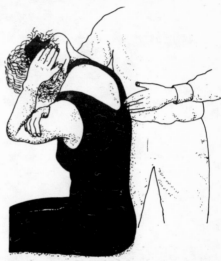

Above *assisted isometric contraction of erector spinae muscles on left side of upper back*

Left *isometric contraction of erector spinae muscles of left side of the upper back — self treatment*

left side is to be treated, the helper, who should be standing behind the seated patient, passes the right hand under the subject's right shoulder, past the front of the neck and rests the hand on the left shoulder. This allows a good deal of leverage to be applied to bending forwards and sideways as well as to rotation of the trunk to the right. Once positioned, all other features (breathing etc.) are as above.

Muscles involved:

Mid and lower back Erector spinae (including Longissimus dorsi). These are deep spinal supporting muscles of the postural type.

Associated problems:	Back pain and stiffness. Triggers in this muscle group may affect the low back and buttocks or the pelvic region.

Position and method

1. Lie on your unaffected side about six inches from the edge of a bed or table, facing the edge. Your upper arm should be taken behind your body and allowed to hang freely, whilst your lower arm should be taken forward from your body, thus rotating your upper trunk towards the ceiling. Turn your head as far as it can comfortably go towards the ceiling. Carry forward your upper leg and let it hang over the side of the bed, (or table), whilst your lower leg is flexed at hip and knee and rests on the edge of the bed or table with your knee just over the edge. Thus your body is twisted in such a way as to take your pelvis one way and your shoulders another. Full relaxation should be achieved so that your leg hanging over the edge is placing a degree of stretch on the muscles of your low back on that side.

2. Now lift that leg an inch or so, as a slow, deep breath is taken. This is held for 7-10 seconds and then released as your leg is slowly, without sudden movements, allowed to hang further down. After some 10-15 seconds of this, repeat the measure using deep breathing and a slight raising of your leg to produce contraction against

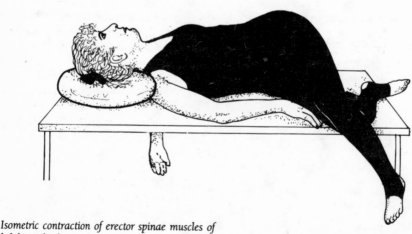

Isometric contraction of erector spinae muscles of left lower back

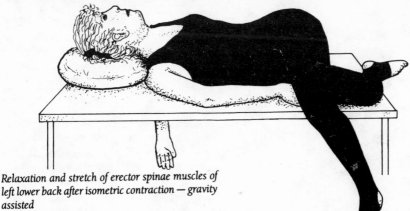

Relaxation and stretch of erector spinae muscles of left lower back after isometric contraction — gravity assisted

gravity's counterpressure. This may be applied to both sides, in turn, for general MET release of the Erector spinae muscles of the mid to low back.

Gravity is such an efficient counterforce in this position that little is to be gained by anyone assisting by providing other forms of restraint, for example by hand pressure.

Muscle involved:	Quadratus lumborum. This is largely a postural muscle which has side bending actions.
Associated problems:	Difficulty in bending sideways and general low back pain and stiffness. Trigger points noted in the waist area are associated with pain in this region, the lower ribs and the crest of the pelvis.

Position and method

1. Stand with your legs 18 inches apart and bend sideways, away from the shortened side, making sure that there is no bending forwards or backwards. Your head should be facing forwards.

2. Having bent sideways as far as is com-

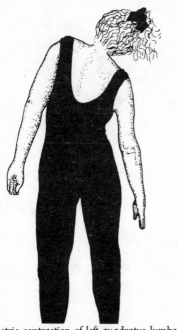

Isometric contraction of left quadratus lumborum muscle

fortable, simultaneously take your trunk an inch or so towards the upright, at the same time looking upwards towards the ceiling out of the corner of your eyes and breathing in deeply. Hold this for a period of 7–10 seconds and then release the breath, turn your eyes towards the floor and relax your muscles, allowing the bend to take your back further towards the floor.

The movement of your eyes automatically tenses your back muscles, preparing them for movement, and this, combined with the breathing and the slight raising of your trunk towards the midline, serves to contract the appropriate muscles against the counterpressure of gravity.

On release, and whilst allowing the muscle to stretch out, breathe in and out several times, very deeply. The stretch position should be held for at least as long as the contraction.

Repeat several times or until no further gain is noted. Repeat on other side if necessary.

Muscles involved:	Middle fibres of trapezius, rhomboids. These lie between your spine and shoulder blade, acting to move this and stabilize it.
Associated problems:	Pain on the inner border of the shoulder blade and between the shoulder blades. Many trigger points are located in these muscles affecting the regions above, below and to the sides.

Position and method

1. Seated. Your arm on the side with most discomfort is taken across your chest so that your hand grasps the area between your neck and shoulder. The angle of this may vary slightly depending upon which muscle fibres are involved. Thus the arm position should be varied until tension is noted in the area of pain.

2. To produce counterpressure grasp with your other hand the elbow of the arm which is reaching across your chest.

3. A deep breath should be taken and this should induce a feeling that the painful area is being stretched by this movement. At the same time you should push the elbow of your arm on the painful side back towards that side, and the shoulder blade towards the spine, using only 25 per cent of the strength available, whilst this is fully resisted. This is held for 5-7 seconds and then gently released as the breath is exhaled.

4. Your arm then should be taken further across your chest to increase the degree of stretch on the tight muscles at the back, ensuring that your shoulder blade is stretched away from your spine. A slight rounding of your back may enhance the

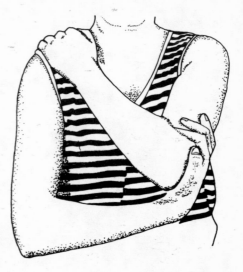

localization of forces at the painful site. Repeat this several times in order to produce relaxation of the tight muscles.

If someone is assisting in this, then they could help by holding the elbow of the arm which is producing the stretch, restraining this as the contractile force is applied when the elbow is pushed back towards the painful side, and the shoulder blade towards the spine. All other aspects of the exercise remain the same.

Muscle involved:	Iliopsoas. This muscle runs obliquely downwards, inside the abdominal cavity from the front surfaces of the upper four lumbar vertebrae to insert in the upper leg. It is a powerful hip and trunk flexor.

Associated problems:

A wide range of problems are associated with psoas contraction, including low back and sciatic pain, distortion of the low back, abdominal pain and discomfort, and groin discomfort.

The lumbar curve may be reversed if the contraction is double-sided (i.e. involving both psoas muscles). This means that instead of a back which curves inwards at the waist, the lower vertebrae could be bowing outwards, giving a characteristic stooped appearance.

If only one psoas is contracted, there may be a twisted and half-stooping posture, typical of 'lumbago'.

Position and method

1. Stand next to the edge of a table with your coccyx area just touching the edge. Bend the knee of the unaffected side and grasp it with both hands, bringing it up towards your chest.

Now sit right on the edge of the table, then roll backwards to lie on it, so that the leg on the affected side is hanging free and the other is held to your chest. This places stretch on the iliopsoas on the affected side. If psoas is shortened, your thigh will be elevated from the horizontal. If it were normal and relaxed it would lie parallel with the table surface.

If your lower leg is not hanging freely but appears to be fairly elevated, thus keeping your leg moderately straight, then the rectus femoris muscle requires treatment before psoas. This is described on page 89.

If your lower leg is hanging fairly freely

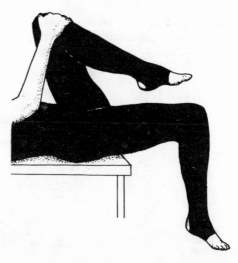

Isometric contraction of right iliopsoas muscle — gravity assisted

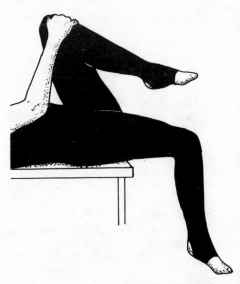

Above *relaxation and stretch of right iliopsoas muscle after gravity assisted isometric contraction*

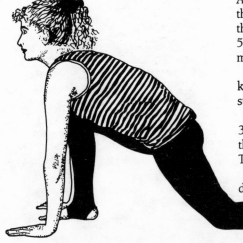

and your upper leg (thigh) is elevated from the horizontal, then proceed with self-treatment. The knee of the free hanging leg should be lifted towards the ceiling by an inch or so, as a deep breath is taken in. Hold the breath for a period of 5-7 seconds before releasing. At this stage your leg should be allowed to hang freely again, for about 10 seconds, thus stretching the psoas. Repeat this sequence several times.

If both psoas muscles are involved then the same method is applied to the other leg. Keep all movements slow to avoid upsetting the psoas again.

2. Kneel on the floor with one knee on the floor as far back as possible from the trunk of the body, and the foot of your other leg on the floor in front of your trunk.

Contraction of the iliopsoas on the side of the kneeling leg is achieved by pressing the back knee downwards and forwards against the floor (without movement taking place) as your pelvis is pushed strongly forwards. As this is done, tension should be felt in the thigh of the kneeling leg. At the same time the breath should be taken in and held for 5-7 seconds, as this contraction is maintained.

Release the breath, and try to take your knee a little further back from your body, stretching the psoas on that side.

Repeat the whole sequence several times.

3. Lying face downwards on the floor, bend the knee on the side of the affected psoas. The other remains outstretched.

Place a small cushion under your abdomen to prevent over-arching forwards.

Place a firm cushion under the thigh of your bent leg so that it is held backwards from your body, placing stretch on the psoas. Inhale and hold your breath, and at the same time push your thigh firmly downwards against the cushion. Hold for 10 seconds and release the effort as the breath is released. Increase the thickness of the pillow under the front of your thigh, thus increasing the stretch on the psoas. Repeat several times.

Stretching the left psoas

Muscle involved:	Rectus abdominis. This is a major abdominal muscle running down the front of your body which is involved in movement, support and stability of the area.
Associated problems:	A variety of trigger points are found in this region when tense, and these can produce pain which mimics many organ problems, including gall bladder and stomach conditions. These muscles are strained when posture is poor and the abdomen is chronically distended.

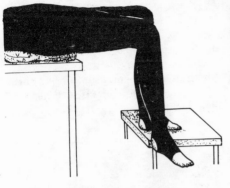

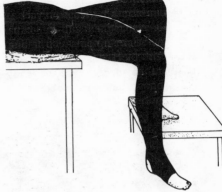

Isometric contraction of rectus abdominis muscle on right side — gravity assisted

Relaxation and stretch of right rectus abdominis muscle after contraction

Position and method

1. Lie on your back on a table with your buttocks right on the edge and both legs over the edge. The foot on your unaffected side should be resting on a stool or chair so that your knee is bent and your leg comfortable. Place a cushion under the buttock on the affected side to raise it slightly, and your leg on that side should hang freely, unsupported. This leg should be lifted slightly, an inch or so, as a deep breath is taken in and held for 5-7 seconds.

As you release the breath, your free hanging leg should be allowed to hang further and to thus stretch the abdominal muscles. Repeat a few times. The same procedure should be repeated on the other leg 3-5 times. This action will release the low end of the muscle.

2. For the other end to be affected, lie on

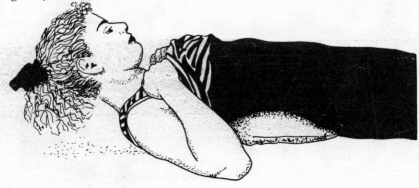

your back with a cushion under your middle back, arching it upwards. Your legs should be straight out, with your arms to the side.

Take a deep breath at the same time as your head and shoulders are rolled gently upwards placing strain on the abdominal muscles. The amount of lift required of the head and shoulders is minimal, only an inch or so. This lift is held for 3–5 seconds and then slowly released, as your breath is exhaled. Repeat several times.

Both ends of the muscle will benefit from MET and they should be treated one after the other.

Muscles involved:

Oblique abdominal muscles. These are postural muscles involved in the maintenance of position of the spine and abdominal organs.

Associated problems:

These muscles are under severe stress, and contract when the abdomen protrudes chronically. Trigger points found in these muscles can produce local pain which mimics internal disease; for example, appendicitis.

Position and method

1. Lie on the floor, on your back, with a cushion under your waist to arch your stomach upwards. Place your hands, clasped, behind your neck. Take a deep breath and simultaneously raise your trunk at least 6 inches until your shoulder blades

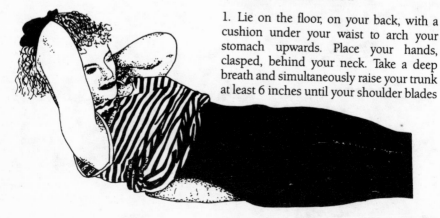

almost leave the surface. A half twist should be introduced, as though you were going to raise your trunk while aiming your nose at the knee of one leg. This will effectively contract the oblique abdominals on the side towards which the twist is taking place.

2. Hold the slight lift and your breath for 5–7 seconds and then release both and lie back over the cushion. Allow relaxation to take place and the abdominal muscles to stretch freely over the arch produced by the cushion under your back.

3. Repeat the contraction several times more in one direction, before using the twist of your trunk to involve the other oblique abdominals in a similar series of contractions on the other side. Increase the size of the cushion if the abdominals are not felt to be well stretched by the relaxation period between contractions. It is important that this rest phase should last at least as long as the contractions. The cushion under your waist should not be under the pelvis at all but in the hollow above it.

Muscle involved: Ligament of the sacro-iliac joint. This lies between the sacrum at the base of the spine and the ilium, the large bone in the pelvis. It is a supporting structure, but has a certain amount of 'give' which is vital for free walking and pelvic movement.

Associated problems: This region is plagued with mechanical stress and this may involve chronic pain in either the sacro-iliac or iliolumbar ligaments.

Position and method

1. Lie on your back on the floor. (A bed may be too soft.) Your knee and hip on the affected side should be bent fully and grasped in both hands, one on top of the other. Your lower hand should draw the knee towards and across the midline (called adduction) and the other pulls the knee towards your chest. The correct positioning will vary according to the point at which the most discomfort is noted in the sacro-iliac region, and where adduction (the pull towards and across the midline) is most resistant, which is the position used for treatment.

2. As you breathe in, your knee should be pushed back towards the side, against the counterpressure of your hand, using only slight pressure. This is held for 10 seconds

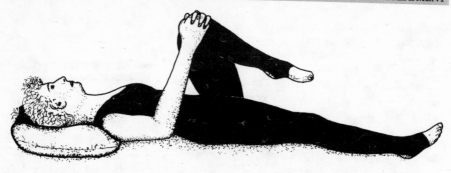

Isometric contraction for sacroiliac ligaments of left side

before being released, at the same time as the breath is released.

When fully relaxed, your leg should be taken slightly further into adduction in the direction of resistance. This can be uncomfortable and should be done slowly.

3. Maintaining maximum adduction and flexion towards the chest, again introduce an isometric contraction against the hold-ing hand(s) on your knee, whilst breathing as before. Repeat the sequence 3 or 4 times.

If someone is assisting then they may provide the counterpressure by placing their hands on the knee of the flexed leg. Whilst counterpressure is sustained in this way, effort to return the leg to the side is made, using only a small degree of effort.

Assisted isometric contraction for sacroiliac ligaments of left side

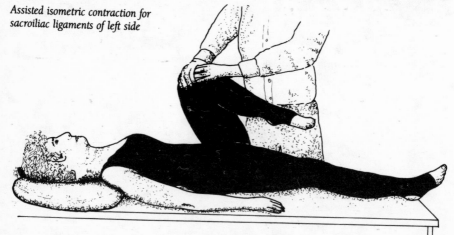

All other factors are as above.
See the section on self-mobilization for other methods of treating the sacro-iliac joint, one of the back's great trouble makers.

Muscle involved:	Serratus anterior and posterior and pectoralis (lower fibres) and other muscles associated with respiration.
Associated problems:	Breathing function and rib mobility restrictions.

Position and method

1. Seated. Rest your open hands on your lower ribs so that your fingers are pointing forwards, with thumbs stretched backwards around your ribs. Breathe deeply in and then exhale completely, compressing the ribs forcefully with your hands so that all air is squeezed from the lungs, leaving them like empty bellows.

At this point, maintain the counter-pressure of your hands, which are pushing towards each other, at the same time as beginning an inhalation which this counterpressure prevents. Your chest is trying to expand; your hands prevent it from doing so. After 5 seconds of this, release the pressure and allow a full deep breath to take place. Breathe normally and deeply several more times before exhaling completely as above and repeating the exercise.

2. Conversely, the muscles may be relaxed isometrically by taking a very deep breath and holding this inhalation, with the chest fully expanded. After 10 to 15 seconds exhale completely and then take several normal and several deep breaths, before repeating the breath holding.

Note: you may feel dizzy, so do not rise too quickly from the sitting position. Do not use this method if suffering from hypertension (high blood pressure) or a cardiac condition.

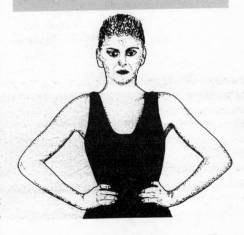

If assisance is available then counter-pressure can be localized by the hands of the helper to restrict an attempted inhalation, thus highlighting selected areas of the rib cage for isometric contraction.

This can be done lying on your back or sitting, with the helper applying counter-pressure as in the first method above or on other areas of the chest as inhalation is attempted after complete exhalation.

Muscles involved:	Levator ani and gluteus maximus. These lie at the base of the spine and buttocks.
Associated problems:	A painful coccyx, which makes sitting uncomfortable, may be associated with unnatural tension in these muscles.

Position and method

1. Lie face downwards, place your hands on your buttocks at the level of your anus, just lateral to this, on the large muscle mass. Your legs should be rotated so that your heels are as far apart as possible whilst your toes remain touching.
2. Contract the muscles of your buttocks, thus squeezing them together, with less than

Isometric contraction of gluteus maxims and levator ani muscles for relief of coccyx pain — counterforce is same muscle on other side — i.e. they are pressing against each other

full strength (i.e. about 25 per cent) and maintain this for 10 seconds before releasing. This isometric contraction consists of the two muscle masses pressing against each other. Repeat this several times.

If this fails to improve your painful coccyx, then the cause may lie in piriformis muscle contraction which is dealt with next.

In most cases one or other of these methods will relieve the condition, but in rare instances the problem lies in the bony structures which would require expert attention.

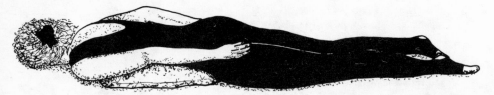

Assistance from someone else in this exercise could involve resting their hands on your buttocks during and after the contraction as described above. This enables a monitoring of the relaxation phase and is of some help, although the mechanics of the method do not require counterpressure in this instance.

Muscle involved:	Piriformis Areas: Hips, buttocks. This muscle is strategically placed so as to be capable of causing pressure on the sciatic nerve, which passes under, over or through it if it is unnaturally shortened. The muscle runs from the side of the sacrum to the back of the hip.
Associated problems:	Contraction of the piriformis which is involved in turning the hip outwards can result in pain along the distribution of the sciatic nerve, i.e. all down the leg, as well as numbness. It can also cause local pain and discomfort in the hip and buttock region, sometimes causing coccygeal pain, or pain in the groin area.

Position and method

There are several methods of dealing with a tight piriformis in self-treatment.

1. Lie on the floor with the foot of your affected leg resting on a stool or chair, press downwards gently with the heel of that foot, at the same time as pulling the knee of that leg towards yourself.

This movement is resisted by placing your hand(s) against your knee. Hold the isometric contraction for 10 seconds before releasing slowly.

The contraction involves the quadriceps muscle on the front of the thigh. This is an antagonist of the piriformis muscle and its isometric contraction produces reciprocal inhibition of the piriformis. Stretch the piriformis by rotating your foot and leg inwards and holding this for up to ten seconds, after the isometric contraction. Repeat.

2. Lie face downwards. Your leg on the side

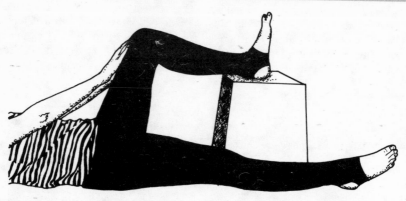

Assisted isometric contraction of the antagonist of the left piriformis muscle

to be treated should be bent at the knee and your lower leg allowed to fall outwards, rotating your upper leg internally.

When all the slack has been taken out, (i.e. complete relaxation), your foot and lower leg should be moved slightly towards the upright, an inch or so, and held for 15-20 seconds before being released and being allowed to fall outwards, again into rotation, for a further 15-20 seconds. Repeat this sequence several times.

The contraction against gravity, when your lower leg is raised slightly, involves the piriformis itself and the subsequent increased stretch effect is therefore the result of post isometric relaxation.

3. (not illustrated) Lie face upwards, right against a wall, with your affected side away from the wall.

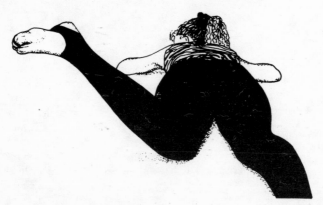

Gravity assisted isometric contraction left piriformis muscle

Bend both knees and touch the area of the affected piriformis with that side's hand. This is done purely to make sure that no increase in tension occurs during the exercise which follows.

Breathe in and push the knee of your *unaffected* side against the wall. The breath should be held for 10 seconds. The degree of push should be quite strong and your monitoring hand should ensure that no increase in tension is felt on the side of the affected piriformis.

After letting go of your breath, and the effort, rest for a period of 10 seconds and then repeat.

The contraction of one piriformis (which happens as your unaffected leg is pushed towards the wall) produces a variation on reciprocal inhibition, relating to what occurs when you walk. Unless one piriformis relaxes as the other contracts during locomotion, you would not walk freely. In this way you can 'make' the tense piriformis relax by forcibly contracting its opposite number.

After this particular technique, use either methods 1 or 2 on page 88 to further stretch the muscle, or lying on your back, cross the affected side leg over the straight other leg so that the foot rests on the floor, alongside the extended knee. Then with your hand push the knee of the affected side leg towards the unaffected side until you feel a stretch behind your hip. Hold for 5 to 10 seconds as the piriformis is stretched in this way before repeating an isometric method (1 or 3 above).

Muscle involved:	Rectus Femoris. This runs down the front of the thigh, on the inner aspect and is a flexor of the knee as well as being a postural muscle.
Associated problems:	Being a postural muscle it may become shortened with stress or dysfunction, often involving knee dysfunction or pain.

Position and method

1. Stand, facing a wall or heavy piece of furniture. The leg to be stretched should be positioned behind your trunk with your knee bent. Hold your leg at the ankle with one hand whilst stabilizing your body against a wall or heavy piece of furniture. Your knee should be bent as far as possible and your thigh stretched backwards.

The isometric contraction is achieved by exerting pressure downwards with your

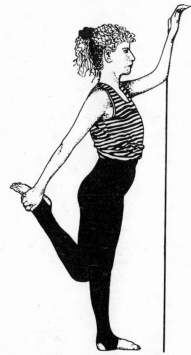

2. If someone is assisting, then lie face downwards. The helper then places a hand under your bent knee and lifts your leg so that the front of your hip is being painlessly stretched.

By resting your lower leg against the arm so that your foot is around the helper's shoulder level, it is possible to exert pressure against your lower leg, further bending your knee to its limit (taking your heel towards your buttock).

When your knee and hip are at their greatest painless stretch in this position, the foot of the treated leg should be pushed against the upper arm or shoulder of the helper (i.e. try to straighten the leg) so that an isometric contraction develops.

Not a great deal of effort is subsequently required to achieve release of the affected muscle by post isometric relaxation. As relaxation is introduced after a 10 second contraction, your knee and hip should be further flexed to introduce more stretch.

lower leg against the hand holding your ankle. As you do this take a deep breath and hold it for 5-7 seconds, until it is slowly released at the same time as the downward pressure of your lower leg is eased.

After relaxation, extend your thigh further behind your body and bring your heel towards your buttock, so stretching rectus femoris on the front of your thigh and repeat the sequence several more times.

Repeat this sequence three or four times.

| **Muscles involved:** | Hamstrings. These are semimembranosus, gracilis semitendinosus and biceps femoris and are postural supporting muscles lying at the back of the thigh. |
| **Associated problems:** | Pain in the leg and low back; pain in the buttock region. |

Position and method

1. Stand with your foot of the leg to be treated on a stool or bench, with your knee straight. The bench provides the resistant counterpressure against which the isometric contraction is achieved.

The contraction develops as you lean your trunk forward, whilst taking a deep breath which should be held for 7–10 seconds. As you exhale the forward lean should be reduced, and when relaxation is fully established, after a few seconds, the forward lean should be taken further, until the maximum stretch is again achieved. This should be further than the previous stretch. Additional stretch is achieved by moving your leg forward on the bench.

2. A second method can be used lying on your back with the aid of a strap which you pass around your lower leg below the knee.

Lying on your back, your leg needing treatment should be straight out, and held as high as possible to achieve maximum stretch painlessly.

If the test for shortened hip flexors (psoas etc.) as described on pages 43 and 44 indicate that these flexors are short, then the hamstring stretch should be performed

with your other leg, flexed at hip and knee and foot flat on the table or floor. If no hip flexor shortening is found, the hamstring stretch should be performed with your other leg straight.

Isometric contraction of hamstring muscles on the left

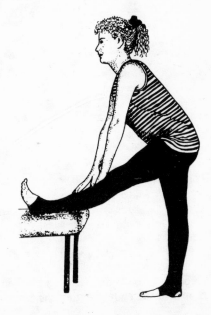

The counterpressure of the isometric contraction is provided by the pushing of your lower leg against the strap, knee held straight, for 7-10 seconds during deep inhalation.

As your breath is released your leg should be relaxed. After this your leg should be taken higher (all the while keeping it straight, as any bend nullifies stretch on the hamstrings).

Having again fully extended your leg, a further isometric contraction is started against the strap's restraint. Repeat this several times. If assistance is available the strap is unnecessary; the hands of the helper can provide the counterpressure needed, with your leg extended.

Muscles involved:

Iliotibial band and tensor fascia lata. This band of fascia and muscle runs from above the hip to below the knee on the outer aspect of the thigh. It is an important postural band.

Associated problems:

Postural problems, recurrent low back and knee problems and pain in the hips, legs and buttocks. These tissues are involved in stabilizing the pelvis as well as in moving the leg outwards (abduction).

Position and method

1. Lie on your side on a table, with your hips close to the end. Your upper leg, which is to be treated, hangs down over the edge, your lower leg being flexed at the knee and hip, and resting. Lying relaxed with your upper leg hanging down in this way places stretch on the shortened tissues.

Isometric contraction is introduced against gravity by raising your leg some 1 or 2 inches and holding this for 15-20 seconds. As this is released your leg should be able to stretch further towards the floor,

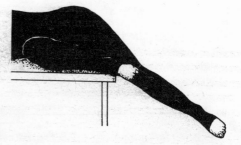

Self treatment isometric contraction for iliotibial band and tensor fascia lata (left side) — gravity assisted

this position being held for 15-20 seconds.

Repeat the seqeunce several more times.

If assistance is available, the counter-pressure against which your leg presses upwards on contraction, can be provided by a helping hand.

2. Otherwise, lie face upwards with your non-treated leg bent at the knee and your treated leg taken across your body, so that your treated leg lies under your bent leg, stretched out towards the opposite side of your body. This places maximum stretch on the fibres on the outer side of your leg. Counterpressure can be provided by a helper's hand. The other hand rests on the pelvis on the treated side, to stabilize this during the isometric contraction, which is produced as an attempt is made to take the extended and adducted leg, back towards its own side.

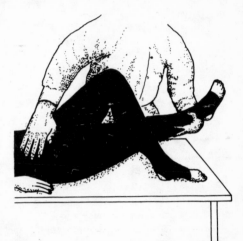

Hold this for 7-10 seconds before release, and a further stretch across the body followed by repetition of the ma-noeuvre several more times. Use breath holding synchronized with the effort, which should be much less than maximum force.

Muscles involved:	Adductors of the thigh, including pectinius, adductors brevis and longus. These lie on the internal aspect of the thighs, and draw the leg inwards and across the body (adduction).
Associated problems:	Limitation in the free movement of the leg. These are postural muscles involved in pelvic stability.

Position and method

1. Sit on the floor, with your feet together and knees as far apart as possible. Your hands should be rested on the inner aspect of your knees, and pressure should be made with your hands to take your thighs out-wards as far as possible. Isometric con-traction is produced by your knees pressing inwards against unyielding counterpressure from your hands on the knees.

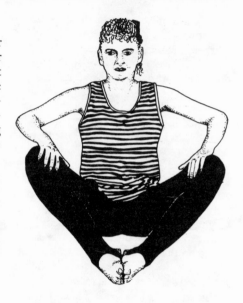

Note: It may be more comfortable to cross your arms as you allow the hands to provide counterpressure against the knees (i.e. left hand on right knee and vice versa).

After the contraction, which should be held for 5-7 seconds, the pressure inwards should be released and your legs may now be able to travel further apart (with your feet always together flat on the floor).

Repeat the sequence several more times.

A helper could provide counterpressure in this position, in which case you could be lying on your back. All other elements remain the same.

2. It is possible to simply separate both knees whilst lying on your back and allow gravity to act as a separating counter-pressure which is slightly overcome by a movement of the flexed knees of about an

inch towards the midline. This position should be held together with an inhaled breath, for about 20 seconds. The longish period of time relates to the lesser counter-force being used in this method.

On relaxation your legs should be allowed to fall apart again to reach maximum separation and stretch of the adductors.

Repeat this several times.

Muscle involved:	Soleus. This lies in the calf.
Associated problems:	Pain in the tendon behind the ankle (achilles tendon) and discomfort in the foot, especially under the arch.

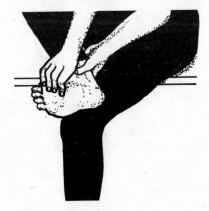

Isometric contraction of soleus muscle on the right

Position and method

1. Sit with one foot on the floor, the leg of the affected foot should be crossed over, so that its heel rests just above the knee of your other, resting leg.
2. Grasp with one hand your leg to be treated, just above the ankle, to stabilize it. With your other hand pull foot into dorsi-flexion, (i.e. the foot is bent upwards at the ankle.)

Usually, one side or the other of the tendon behind your ankle is more sensitive, so your foot should be so positioned as to introduce maximum stretch on that aspect (i.e. turning your foot slightly inwards or outwards as the flexion upwards of the ankle is performed).
3. When maximum stretch is felt in the appropriate muscles, a counterpressure of only moderate force should be exerted by

your foot by attempting to push it straight against unyielding resistance from your hand, for 7-10 seconds.

After relaxation there should be some release of tension, allowing a further up-ward stretch of your foot.

Repeat the sequence as above.

If assistance is available, then counter-pressure can be offered by the helper's hand in precisely the same manner as in self-treatment. This is sometimes better achieved in assisted MET by lying face down and flexing your affected leg at the knee. The helper can then stabilize your lower leg with one hand, whilst stabilizing your foot appropriately with the other against resisted effort to flex the foot down-wards (plantar flexion, in which the short muscle is contracted isometrically).

In order to stretch both soleus muscles adopt the test position as shown on page 44, making sure that your heels do not leave the floor as you go into a squat. At the point where they feel they are going to leave the floor you should stop trying to squat, re-maining in that position for ten seconds or so (this produces an isometric contraction of both soleus muscles). After this try to go a little further into the squat. Repetition of this for several minutes on a daily basis will stretch the muscle to its normal length with-in a few weeks. There may be a tendency to feel you are falling forwards as you squat. If so, balance yourself by holding a heavy piece of furniture with one or both hands as you go down with back rounded forwards. These muscles shorten dramatically when high heels are worn.

Muscle involved:

Gastrocnemius.
This lies in the calf at the back of the lower leg.

Associated problems:

Pain in the knee or lower leg.

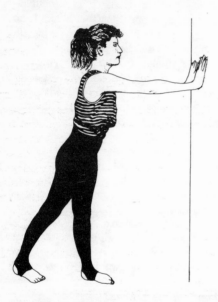

Position and method

1. Stand facing a wall with your hands on the wall as stabilizers. Your affected leg should be taken backwards so that your foot remains flat on the floor and your knee straight. The furthest position backwards from the wall is achieved in this manner, placing maximum stretch on your leg muscles behind your knee. Greater stretch is achieved by pushing your pelvis forwards.

When this has been done, isometric contraction of the appropriate muscle is achieved by pressing your foot against the floor and holding this for 5–7 seconds before releasing pressure.

When released and relaxed, your leg may be able to be taken further backwards and your pelvis pushed further forwards before repetition of the sequence.

Take a deep breath at the beginning of the effort to enhance the effect, releasing your breath at the end of the contraction. A strong pull will be felt in your calf as maximum stretch is achieved.

Repeat until no further stretch can be gained.

Muscles involved:

Extensors of the toes.
These lie in front of the lower leg.

Associated problems:

When these are tight pain is often felt in the front of the lower leg (shin).

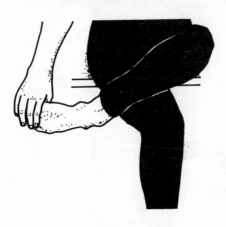

Position and method

1. Sit with your affected leg crossed over the other and by grasping your toes and dorsum (top) of your affected foot, bring it into maximum flexion, stretching the affected muscles.
2. Try to push against this with the muscles of your foot, using a fair degree of strength, for 10 seconds, before relaxing.
3. Repeat three or four times.

Left *treatment of tightness in extensors of the toes using an isometric contraction*

Muscle involved:

Aponeurosis of foot.
This is the area of the sole (plantar surface) of the foot.

Associated problems:

A calcaneal spur often develops when these tissues are tight.

Position and method

1. Cross your affected leg over your other leg in a seated position. Grasp and stabilize your heel with one hand, and steady your toes and lower foot with the other, bringing these into dorsiflexion (i.e. top of foot is

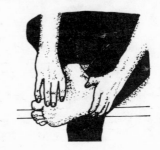

Right *treatment of right aponeurosis of foot*

taken towards the knee) until strong tension is felt under your foot.

2. Your toes and lower foot should then be flexed (bent) against this resistance for 10 seconds before relaxing and repeating three or four times.

Your foot must be kept in dorsiflexion all the time in order to stretch these very fibrous structures.

Muscle involved:	Related to the jaw, i.e. masseter etc. These lie in the jaw and head areas.
Associated problems:	Difficulty in opening mouth, chewing problems, clicking and painful joints in the region, headaches etc.

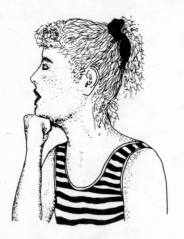

Treatment isometric contraction for jaw muscles

Position and method

1. Sit at a table with the elbow of one hand resting on the table with your cupped hand upwards, into which your chin is placed. (A clenched fist may be used as an alternative.) Your mouth should be opened to its comfortable limit.

Attempt to open your mouth further against this unyielding resistance for 5-10 seconds.

Repeat by relaxing, taking your jaw to its new barrier and repeating the isometric contraction against the counterpressure of your hand. Only minimal force should be used.

This method uses RI for its effect.

2. Open your mouth fully and place two fingers of each hand onto the back lower teeth. Your index and ring fingers are best suited for the manoeuvre. Use these as counterpressure whilst you attempt to close your mouth, using less than 20 per cent of the strength in the muscles of your jaw. Hold the contraction for 5 seconds or so before releasing and attempting to open your mouth further.

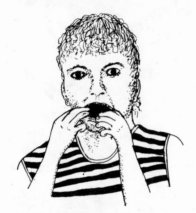

Isometric contraction of jaw muscles

Repeat several times.

Your fingers may be protected against injury from your teeth by wrapping them in a handkerchief.

3. If deviation to one side is noted on opening your mouth, then restriction exists on the side which deviation occurs.

Open your mouth fully and, with your hands, push the deviated side of the jaw towards the normal side and resist for 4–7 seconds, while holding your breath.

Repeat several times.

Alternatively, the muscles of your stretched side may be used to try to pull your jaw 'straight' against hand resistance, for similar lengths of time (i.e. counterpressure is towards the side of deviation).

If help is available, the helper's hands can provide counterpressure in the methods described above. Whichever method is used, after the contraction is ceased there should be some release of tension in the tight muscles and these should be lightly stretched towards a more normal position.

Muscles involved:	Flexors and extensors of the lower arm, biceps and supinator. These are involved in all movements of the lower arm and hand.
Associated problems:	Painful outer or inner aspect of elbow (tennis elbow, golfer's elbow etc.)

Position and method

1. If it is difficult to turn your palm down then your *supinator* is shortened. Sitting with your bent elbow held against the side of your body, lower arm across the front of your body, turn your hand palm downwards, and with your other hand turn it further inwards in that direction, as far as possible, painlessly.

Your other hand should offer counterpressure at your wrist as you attempt isometrically to rotate your wrist towards a palm upwards position. This contraction

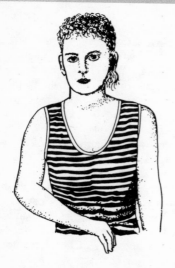

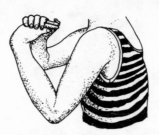

Isometric contraction of extensor muscles of the lower arm

Isometric contraction of supinator muscle of right arm

should be held for 7-10 seconds before being released at which time your hand is taken further into pronation (palm turned downwards). Repeat several times.

2. If it is difficult to bend your wrist downwards (dropped wrist position) or for your fingers to bend, then the *extensors* of your lower arm may be shortened.

Sit with the elbow of your affected arm bent and the inner aspect of your forearm turned towards you, wrist bent, so that your hand is pointing towards your face, palm down.

Using your other hand, flex your affected wrist and fingers as far as possible, before making an effort to extend your wrist against this counterpressure.

On relaxation, increase the degree of flexion in your wrist and fingers before

repeating the exercise. This isometric contraction should be held for 5-7 seconds and repeated as necessary.

Repeat several times after appropriate relaxation and further stretching of the tight joints.

3. If straightening your elbow is difficult, then your *biceps* muscle is probably shortened.

Sit cross-legged and rest your affected elbow on your knee and straighten it as far as possible. Have your extended arm palm upwards where possible, and use your other hand to offer counterpressure on the forearm, against an attempt to bend your elbow. Hold the isometric contraction for 5-7 seconds, before releasing and stretching the arm towards a straighter position.

Alternatively, having extended your arm, with your elbow resting on your knee, bend it and raise your forearm an inch or so, holding this position for 10 seconds or so, with gravity providing the counterpressure. On release, your arm should be able to extend further than previously.

Repeat this several times.

4. If there is pain on the inner aspect of

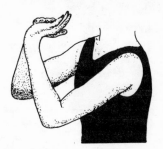

Isometric contraction of flexors of lower arm

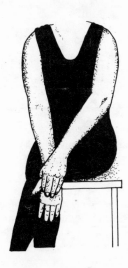

Isometric contraction of the biceps

your elbow then the *flexors* of your forearm may be shortened.

Sit with your elbow bent, palm turned upwards and fingers pointing towards your face. Your other hand should be placed so that there is pressure downwards on the little finger side of your affected palm, pushing this aspect gently further into an outwards rotation of your hand.

The isometric contraction is introduced as your affected hand is moved towards internal rotation. This means that the effort is directed to attempting to turn your palm inwards against the unyielding counter-pressure of your unaffected hand.

The contraction should be held for 5-7 seconds and repeated after appropriate relaxation, after the taking up of the slack in the treated muscle.

Assistance in any of these measures in-

volves replacing the patient's hands with those of a helper, to provide the various directions of counterpressure described above.

5. If there is pain localized in the front of your upper arm several inches below your shoulder joint, this may relate to a shortened *biceps insertion*. Treatment involves moving that arm behind your back and across your body as far as is comfortable. Ensure that your palm is facing downwards.

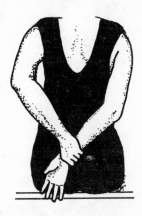

Isometric contraction affecting biceps insertion

With your other hand, take out the slack and fix this at its furthest rotation and gently try to derotate (i.e. turn your palm upwards) against the counterpressure for 10 seconds.

On release, take out more slack by turning your wrist further into pronation and stretch your elbow further (i.e. take it further across towards the opposite side).

Repeat several times.

Isokinetic methods

If any small joint is weak following injury or immobilization, self-help isokinetic methods can be used. A finger, wrist, toe, ankle etc. can be held and partial resistance offered to an attempt to rapidly move it in all available directions, using its own muscles for the effect. Thus, a finger can be held so that whatever it does will be somewhat restrained by the grip; at this point it should be flexed, extended, bent and rotated by its own muscles, against this resistance. The amount of force used should eventually approach the full muscular strength available as long as this does not produce pain.

Initially a 4–5 second series of rapid, resisted movements, involving no more than half available strength is advisable. Subsequent series of movements should build up to greater degrees of effort.

Larger joints are not suitable for self-treatment using this method, although with the assistance of someone else, larger joints such as the knee, elbow etc. can be so treated.

Toning weak muscles

Isotonic contractions can be used in treating larger joints quite easily, where muscle tone is poor and requires attention. Use of weights in lifting represents a basic isotonic resistance to effort. Similar self-help resistance methods can be used. For example, by holding the forearm with the other hand as it bends upwards and thus partially resisting its effort, we are effectively toning up the flexors of the arm.

Any attempt to tone weak muscles should be left until after any tight contracted areas in the vicinity are stretched and loose (using MET or other methods) since it is the tension in these which may be inhibiting and weakening the flaccid muscles which appear to need toning. If attention is paid to the identification and stretching of tight structures first, toning exercises will be seldom needed and will be more successful when they are.

Listed below are a selection of methods based on the work of Dr H.J.A. Schmid of Berne (see page 54) which should be used to tone muscles in the low, mid or upper back as needed *after* appropriate (as determined by tests outlined in Chapter 3) stretching exercises have been performed for some weeks. As tight postural muscles are stretched, the inhibition (weakness) their tension will have been causing to antagonist phasic muscles will be reduced, allowing self-toning of these to occur naturally.

It is only at this stage that active isotonic exercises may be called for.

Gluteus Maximus: This large buttock muscle extends and externally rotates the upper leg and is inhibited if there is a short/tight psoas condition. Tone it if it fails the following test: Lying face down with a pillow under the stomach, bend the knee and lift the thigh off the table (without arching the back). If this is difficult Gluteus maximus needs toning. Tone it by standing at the edge of a table and placing the trunk, from the hips upwards, onto the table with one foot remaining on the floor and the leg of the side of the weak gluteus raised to the horizontal (parallel with the floor). Take care not to over-arch the low back and keep the pelvis flat on the table (no twist) as you try to hold the leg in this position for 8 seconds. Rest and repeat several times (on both sides if both gluteals are weak). Do this twice daily until it is easy.

Gluteus medius and minimus: These lie on the outer side of the pelvis and act as abductors of the leg (they take it out sideways as well as slightly rotating it internally). If the exercise described is difficult then they need toning. They may become weak if piriformis or adductors or hamstrings are tight.

Lie on your side with the side to be exercised upwards. Bend the lower leg at hip and knee to stabilize yourself. Have the upper body tilted forward of the pelvis very slightly (about ten degrees from the upright). Raise the upper leg sideways from the body and hold this for about 8 seconds. Rest and repeat up to five times on each side.

Deltoid: This thick muscle covers the shoulder joint and raises the arm upwards, forwards or backwards or rotates it. It may become weak when trapezius, levator scapulae or pectoralis major are tight and short. When this exercise is done be careful to relax the trapezius muscle which lies between the shoulder and the neck. Stand sideways on to a wall with the side nearest the wall being the side to be treated. Relax the neck/shoulder and push strongly against the wall with the side of your bent elbow. Hold for 8 seconds, relax and repeat up to 5 times.

Rhomboids and lower trapezius: These muscles overlap each other (rhomboids underneath) and lie between the spine and the shoulder blade. They stabilize the shoulder blade and move it to accommodate arm movement. They often become weak when upper trapezius, levator scapulae, spinal erectors or pectoralis major are short and tight.

Sit in a chair with a high back, pressing the lower angle of your shoulder blades downwards and inwards against the back of the chair. Hold this position for 8 seconds, and after a short rest, repeat up to five times. If shoulder problems are chronic do the Rhomboid/lower trapezius exercise first and while holding this position perform the deltoid exercise at the same time.

Note: this assortment of muscle energy techniques is by no means a comprehensive listing of all the possible body areas which may be self-treated. Nor is it a definitive listing of the methods available. Many more exist and will be evolved. The methods are simple and safe; variations may be discovered by the explorer of the system and its opportunities, while the basic ground-rules of muscle energy technique, once grasped, open a wide vista of possible uses.

Many methods in which a practitioner or other person may assist in muscle energy methods have not been included in this book, where the technicalities of these procedures might confuse what is meant to be essentially a series of self-help, first-aid measures aimed at offering relief from pain and common muscle and joint problems.

Causes should always be sought for such problems, for treating the symptoms alone (tight muscles and joints, pain etc.) is never enough.

More detailed discussion of MET and other soft tissue techniques, are to be found in my book *Soft Tissue Manipulation* (Thorsons, 1988). It is suggested that close attention be paid to the methods described in the chapters dealing with self-mobilization and exercise, as these complement the muscle energy procedures described.

Remember to always loosen what is tight and restricted before attempting to tone up weak structures.

Freeing tight joints

Any joint which is restricted in any direction can be self-treated by muscle energy methods.

Take the joint towards its restrictive barrier. Avoid taking it to a point which is painful. Fix it at that point and then either gently try to take it further towards the barrier against resistance, or take it away from the barrier against resistance. Using minimal effort, never allowing pain to occur, hold this for 7–10 seconds. Ease off and relax and then take the joint further towards its barrier. This is muscle energy, a supremely effective, gentle and safe method.

5

Trigger points
and their importance

When muscles are placed under stress due to misuse, strain, postural abuse etc, they have a tendency to develop localized areas which become sensitive and which themselves are the source of discomfort in distant tissues in what are termed 'target areas'.

These localized areas are called trigger points and have been shown by researchers to be the cause of a great deal of pain and other symptoms. It is important that we realize that only those tender, localized areas which under pressure send symptoms to a target area are active trigger points. All other localized sensitive areas are potential trigger points, which may become active should they be irritated in some way (a cold draught, postural, emotional or other physical stress etc.)

Once a point becomes an active trigger, it may vary in the intensity of its symptoms, but it never stops its activity unless and until some physical method is used to deal with it. Triggers in specific muscle areas, in different people, produce symptoms in the same target area in everyone, which makes their identification reasonably easy.

Assessing whether pain results from local or referred (trigger) sources may be accomplished by applying gentle, localized finger pressure to the area where the pain is felt. If the pain gets worse with moderate pressure this indicates that the pain is coming from the place where it is being pressed and therefore is not the result of trigger point activity.

If, however, pressure is applied to a painful area and the pain is not felt to increase, it is safe to assume that the pain is being referred from somewhere else, and reference to a chart of trigger points can give guidance as to where to seek the active trigger requiring attention. Trigger points *always* lie in muscle fibres which have shortened, and these usually, but not inevitably, lie in muscles which are hypertonic. This means they are contracted.

One of the main rules of trigger point removal is that whatever method of initial treatment is used, and there are many, the muscle in which the trigger lies has to be stretched to allow it to reach its normal resting length after such treatment, otherwise the trigger will remain active or will rapidly return to its negative behaviour. Muscle Energy Technique is the easiest and safest way of stretching such muscles.

Once found, trigger points may be treated in several ways, all of which are equally successful, but some of which are more easily applied. Some of these are amenable to self-application. However, before considering how to self-treat trigger points we need to be able to find them.

1. If there is pain or tenderness in a

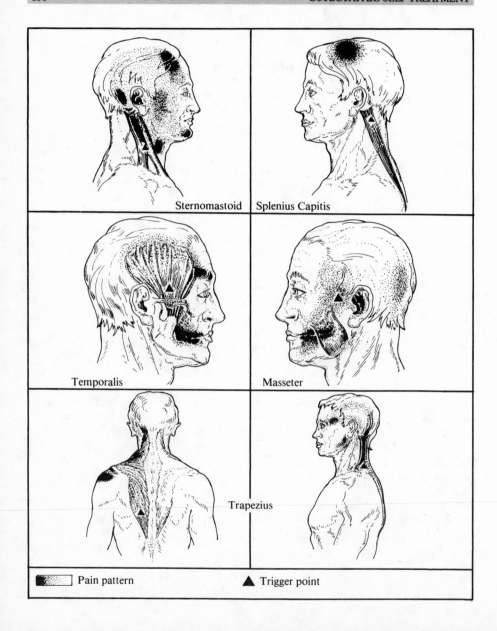

Sternomastoid   Splenius Capitis

Temporalis   Masseter

Trapezius

Pain pattern   ▲ Trigger point

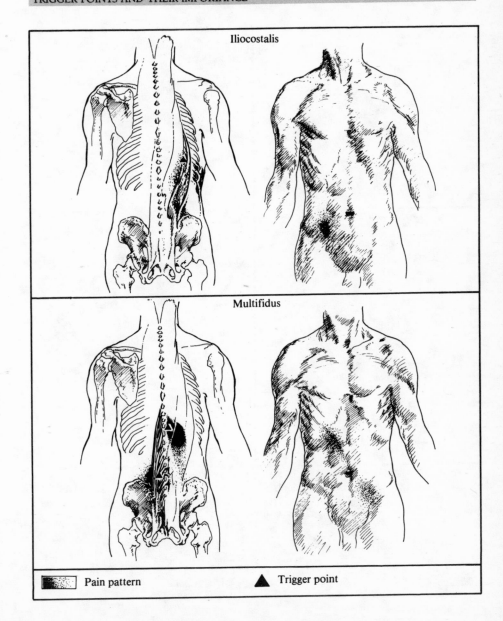

Iliocostalis

Multifidus

Pain pattern   ▲ Trigger point

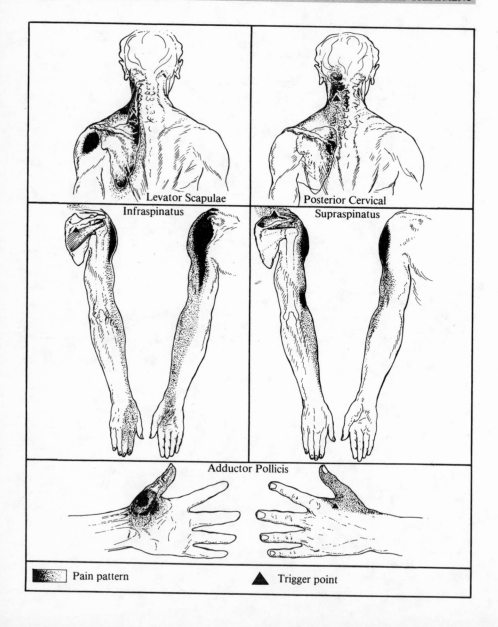

Levator Scapulae

Posterior Cervical

Infraspinatus

Supraspinatus

Adductor Pollicis

Pain pattern   Trigger point

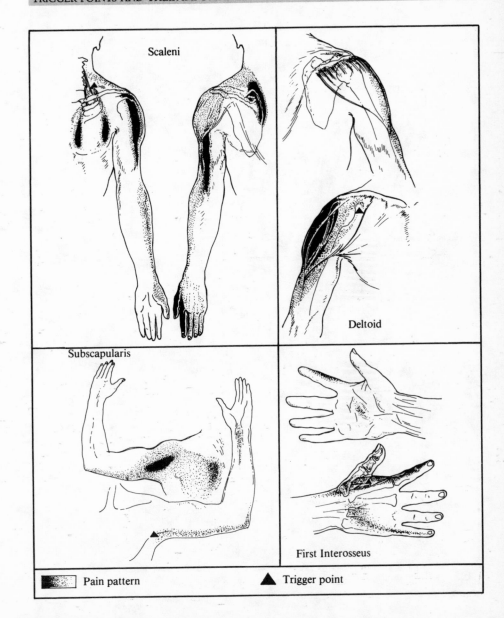

Scaleni

Deltoid

Subscapularis

First Interosseus

Pain pattern ▲ Trigger point

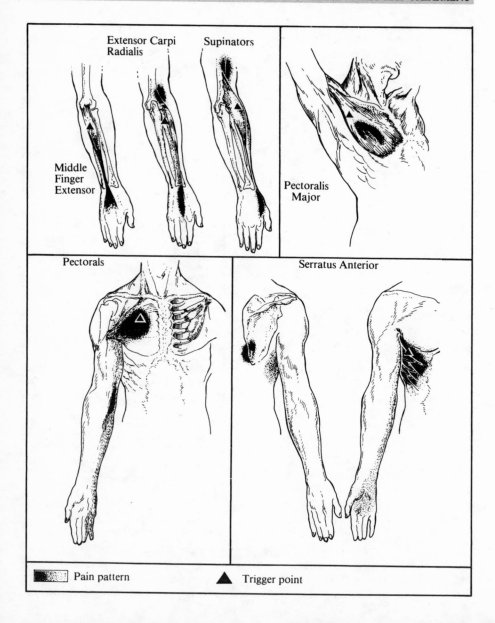

Extensor Carpi Radialis

Supinators

Middle Finger Extensor

Pectoralis Major

Pectorals

Serratus Anterior

◼️▒ Pain pattern   ▲ Trigger point

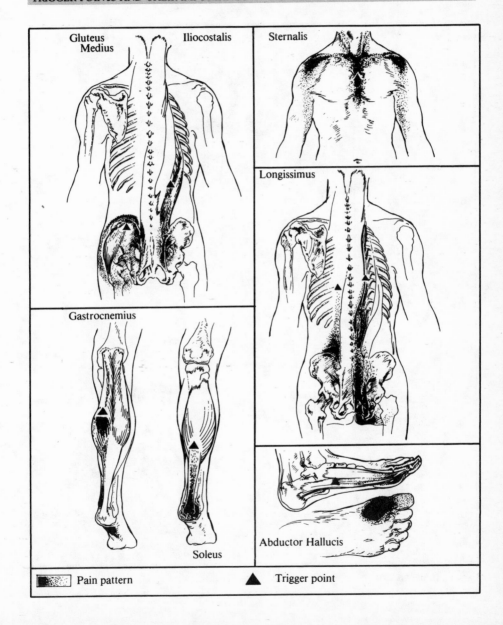

Gluteus Medius

Iliocostalis

Sternalis

Longissimus

Gastrocnemius

Soleus

Abductor Hallucis

Pain pattern   Trigger point

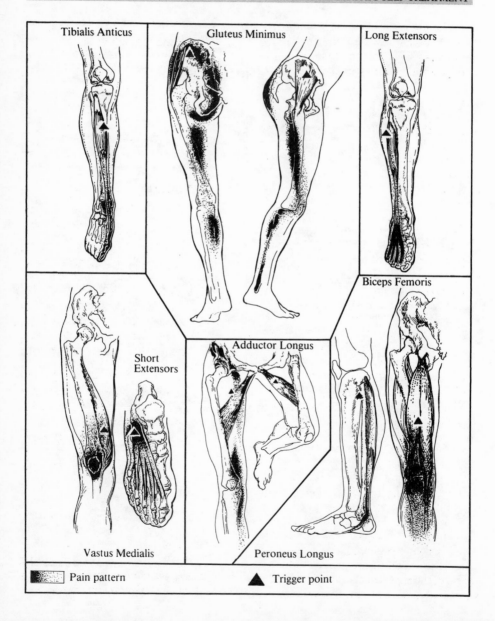

Tibialis Anticus

Gluteus Minimus

Long Extensors

Biceps Femoris

Short
Extensors

Adductor Longus

Vastus Medialis

Peroneus Longus

Pain pattern   Trigger point

particular area of the body, refer to the chart showing common trigger points and their target areas. First apply local pressure of a moderate, but not heavy, nature, to the area of pain.

Does it get worse?

If so, the cause probably does not stem from trigger point activity.

If pressure on a sensitive area, (such as one which had been recurrently or permanently tender for some time) does not increase the degree of local discomfort or pain then trigger point activity may be causing it. Consult the chart of common trigger points and search by diligent pressure and/or squeezing of the appropriate area until a localized sensitive area is found. Stay pressing or squeezing this for some 5 seconds, then note whether this produces increased pain in the target area. If it does, you have found the trigger.

If it does not, or refers somewhere else you have either found a latent (non-active) trigger or a trigger relating to another target area. Search on for the one causing your particular symptom of pain. When this is found proceed according to one or other of the options listed below.

2. If you do not start from the target and work back towards where the trigger may be coming from, as in 1. above, then it is possible to find trigger points by gently probing with fingers or thumb the various tight or aching muscles of the body.

Favourite sites for triggers are the neck and shoulder muscles as well as those of the low back. In searching through the neck muscles, remember to squeeze the tissues between finger(s) and thumb in order to assess them, do not probe with fingers or thumbs over the side or front of the neck. In searching in this way it is common to find localized, slightly hard areas which are quite small (often no bigger than a lentil) but which are sensitive under pressure.

If the pressure or squeeze is maintained for 5 seconds or so, at a reasonably strong level and this is an active trigger, it will begin to send symptoms to an area some distance away (see chart). This is a trigger point.

Treatment of trigger points

1. Direct pressure by finger or thumb on a trigger can be used to decrease its activity. This is performed as follows:

- Press (or squeeze, if the trigger lies in very soft muscle tissue such as that in the upper trapezius muscle (pages 59/60) or in muscles of the neck such as the sternomastoid (page 61/62) where pressure would be unwise) the point until the referred symptoms are noted, and hold this pressure for 5 seconds.
- Ease the pressure off by about 25 per cent or until the referred symptoms are much reduced, for a further 5 seconds.
- Continue this repetition of 5 seconds on, 5 seconds off, for a minute or until, when the pressure is being applied, a marked reduction in the intensity of the referred symptom is felt, as compared with the level at the outset.

2. At this time, pressure or squeezing should stop. The muscle in which the trigger lies now requires stretching.

3. Other methods of trigger point treatment include acupuncture (what has been termed 'dry needling') and this is obviously

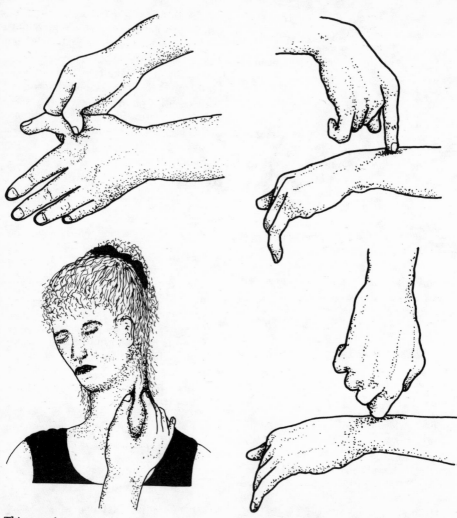

This page how pressure and squeezing of trigger points should be applied

unsuitable for self-treatment.

4. The major researcher into trigger points, Dr Janet Travell, has suggested a method of chilling trigger points prior to stretching the muscles in which they lie. A cold spray using fluoromethane (obtainable from a pharmacy) may be sprayed over the area

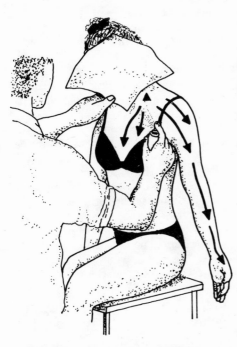

Chilling treatment of trigger point in the scalenus muscles

running from the trigger point to the target area in a series of slow sweeps covering all the muscle tissue between trigger and target. A piece of ice may also be used, directly against the skin, for the same purpose, although this tends to be messy as the ice melts.

An empty soft-drink can filled with water and placed in a freezer for some hours, is a less messy and an even more effective method of chilling the skin between trigger and target. It can then (when filled with ice) be gently rolled along

these tissues for a minute or so, after the pressure method has been used and before, or during, stretching of the muscle, to effectively 'switch off' an active trigger.

Once the area has received this chilling for about 20 seconds (with care taken not to allow blanching or frosting of the skin) the muscle in which the trigger lies requires stretching, just as it would after the pressure method described in 1. above.

5. Muscle Energy Techniques are suggested as an alternative to all the above especially if the trigger is of recent origin. In any case the use of MET after 1. or 3. or 4. above, is an ideal method of achieving the muscle's fully stretched resting length.

If a trigger point has been around for some time, say months or years, then it will almost certainly have become rather fibrosed and hardened. This would be unlikely to just disappear with MET, and after MET would probably require pressure treatment and active stretching as well. If, however, the trigger point is fairly recent and the tissues in which it lies have not yet become 'organized' and fibrosed, it might well respond to muscle energy methods alone.

Trigger points, we must never forget, while causing symptoms themselves, are also caused by something else and unless that cause is eliminated they will return. The cause of a trigger point may result from a joint problem, which would require expert attention. Alternatively, the causes may lie in habitual postural or occupational stresses, which should be identified and corrected or minimized, if possible. Also, causes of trigger points may lie in strain in particular muscles resulting from emotional stresses; these, too, need identification and correction if possible.

Often new triggers develop in target areas, and are therefore known as 'satellite' triggers. These require attention just as much as their 'parent' trigger points. From this it can be seen that simply dealing with a trigger is not enough, although it can provide remarkable relief from symptoms for a while. We need to be able to identify triggers, remove them using safe self-help measures, (pressure, chilling, stretching, MET etc.) and also, if possible, learn to identify causes so that a swift return of symptoms is not noted. It should also be mentioned that Travell's research and that of many others, has shown that trigger points result in symptoms much more complex than pain alone.

I have described this in my book *Instant Pain Control* (Thorsons, 1987) which deals with the trigger point phenomenon, in these words,

> The disturbing effects of trigger points go far beyond the simple production and maintenance of pain. A whole range of symptoms can be produced by triggers via their effect on the nervous system, circulatory function and hormonal balance.
>
> Dr Janet Travell maintains that the high intensity of nerve impulses from an active trigger point can produce, by reflex, vasoconstriction, cutting down the blood supply to specific areas of the brain, spinal cord and nervous system, thus producing any of a wide range of symptoms, capable of affecting almost any part of the body. Such symptoms as disordered vision, disordered respiration, muscle weakness and skin sensitivity, are reported by her as resulting from trigger areas in specific muscles.

Among symptoms reported by Dr Travell and others are the following, all a direct result of trigger point activity, as proved by their disappearance when the triggers were dealt with:

Pain, numbness, itching, over-sensitivity to normal stimuli, spasm, twitching, weakness and trembling of muscles, over- or under-secretion of glands, localized coldness, paleness, redness of tissues; menopausal hot flushes, altered skin texture (very oily, very dry), increased sweat production and, in triggers found in the abdominal and thoracic muscles, halitosis (bad breath), heartburn, vomiting, nausea, distension, nervous diarrhoea and constipation.

Travell also reports symptoms of hysteria which disappear with successful trigger point work.

Rules of self-treatment of trigger points are

1. Treat triggers only to ease pain. Other symptoms, as listed above, may be the result of other causes and a competent diagnosis is needed.
2. Only use trigger point self-treatment from a first-aid point of view. If the pain does not ease, or if it eases and returns, consult a qualified osteopath or chiropractor, as other factors such as joint dysfunction may be maintaining the trigger.
3. Never treat a trigger which lies near or on a swelling, lump, inflamed area etc.
4. Never treat a trigger point which lies on a mole, scar, wart or varicose vein.
5. Never treat a trigger point which lies on a woman's breast.
6. A pregnant woman should never be

treated without medical approval.

7. Take professional advice before using trigger point work in anyone with a diagnosis of cancer or rheumatoid arthritis.

8. Although trigger points are often the same as acupuncture points, never use a needle to self-treat or to treat anyone else, unless you are qualified to do so.

9. Follow the guidelines, given above, for treatment. For example, use only moderate and intermittent pressure, stop when the pain eases or after one minute.

Because *some* pressure helps, it does not follow that *more* will be better. **Never overtreat.** If no response is noted when following the advice given then take professional advice.

10. Always try to discover the causes of trigger points, such as posture, wrong use of the body, occupation, nutritional inadequacy, stress etc.

MET and trigger points

If a muscle contains a trigger point, it is not capable of reaching its normal resting length. Apart from the disruption which the trigger point will be causing to normal function, this imbalance in the muscle can cause problems for other muscles (its antagonists) and the joint(s) to which it relates. Use of MET, as described in the chapters dealing with that most useful of methods, should therefore be used either alone (in recently active triggers) or in combination with pressure, chill and stretch, or acupuncture (not for self-treatment) methods. All that is necessary is that the muscle be asked to perform a series of isometric contractions, followed by gentle stretching of the muscle in the periods between these contractions.

Follow the guidelines in the chapters on MET as to how to achieve the best results, using breathing accompaniment and repetition of the procedure, until no further gain is noted. Never use more than moderate effort with MET and *ensure that the area of the muscle in which the trigger point lies is contracting during the isometric procedure.*

After full stretch is achieved, gently probe or squeeze the area again and note whether the referred symptoms are now gone or much reduced. They should be. Treat the area with respect for some days as muscles which have been disturbed in this way are sensitive and easily upset by overactivity, strain or chills.

Pressure on inaccessible trigger points: the tennis ball trick

Where it is difficult to find a comfortable way of applying pressure to a trigger point or to a tight, tender muscle, it is possible to use a simple strategy which harnesses the properties of a tennis ball, or two. If the area or point is on the back, place a tennis ball on a carpeted floor and lie back onto it so that the tennis ball is just pressing onto the point. It is possible to vary the degree of weight placed on the ball so that deeper or lighter pressure can be sustained for appropriate periods, as described earlier in this chapter.

A similar degree of controlled pressure can be obtained by screwing a rubber doorstop into a doorframe, (or other suitably secure structure) at a height which allows you to stand in front of it,

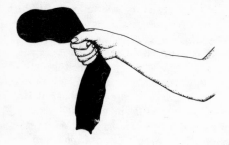

so that pressure can be obtained against chronically tight structures or trigger points simply by leaning against it.

Spinal massage with two tennis balls

If both sides of the spine require pressure simultaneously, as in marked stiffness, two tennis balls may be placed in tandem, so to speak, by stuffing them into the toe of a sock and then tying them securely in position. By lying on these two balls so that the bony prominence of your spine (spinous process) falls between them and a ball rests on each side of your spine, it is not difficult to alter the pressure and even to perform spinal massage by gently moving up and down, so that the balls roll alongside your spine, applying their pressure to the tense tissues.

Self-massage of areas such as the back of your shoulder, or your buttock muscles, is easily accomplished in the same manner, using one or two balls depending on the size of the area requiring soft even pressure.

It is suggested that for general loosening up of tight muscles, you should use a tennis ball (or two) in this fashion for not less than two and not more than five minutes.

For trigger points, of course, a minute is usually adequate using the on-off pressure methods, described above.

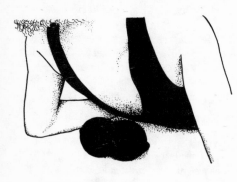

Golf-ball massage for the feet

To massage the tight tissues which are often found under the arches of your feet (commonly associated with painful fallen arches and heel-'spurs'), a similar strategy

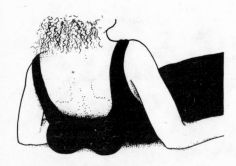

This page *spinal massage with two tennis balls*

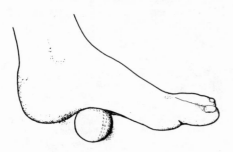

Golf ball massage for the feet

may be employed, but this time using a golf ball.

Sitting in an upright chair place the golf ball onto a carpeted floor and rest the sole of your foot onto it. By rolling your foot up and down and controlling the degree of downwards pressure, a noticeable relaxation of these tight fascial and muscular structures can be achieved.

Regular daily exercise of this sort, should not create more than mild discomfort, but do not be tempted to overdo things at any one session as bruising can result.

Keep pressure tolerable and movement gentle and slow.

Whichever method you find most useful in applying pressure to trigger points, or tight structures, remember that afterwards it is most important that the muscles be stretched, and the the best way of doing this is to incorporate the Muscle Energy Techniques which are described in Chapters 1, 2, 3 and 4.

6

Self-mobilization methods

Muscle Energy Techniques, as outlined in previous chapters, provide us with an excellent series of methods for relaxation and stretching of specific tight, shortened, contracted and painful muscles. But in addition to this, as muscles relating to particular joints are thus loosened, the joints themselves become more mobile and improve in their ability to function normally.

Anyone who has attended Yoga classes will recognize certain similarities between the concepts of Muscle Energy Technique, and the methods used by Yoga teachers in assisting people in the attainment of the various postures associated with that system. After adopting an approximation of the posture desired, the student in Yoga is asked to breathe slowly and deeply and to maintain the posture for a minute or two. In some instances, holding of breath is encouraged during part of this period. After a minute or two the student is asked to take a deep breath, release it and, simultaneous with the exhalation, to try to duplicate more accurately the pose being attempted.

Having now looked at Muscle Energy methods, the reader will recognize that by taking up a posture (say sitting with the legs outstretched, trying to reach the toes with the finger tips) and taking the body to the pain-free limit in any given direction; then holding this position, he or she is in fact creating an isometric contraction in which the effort towards the chosen direction is matched by a counterpressure of resistance from his/her tight muscles.

The breathing pattern used in Yoga allows for relaxation to be enhanced, as the physiological response to the multiple isometric contractions involved are engineered in this way. Indeed if we are seeking a method for general stretching and mobilization (as opposed to the specific techniques outlined in the Muscle Energy Technique chapters) we need look no further than Yoga.

It is not difficult to devise a series of exercises or postures in which general mobilization of regions of the body may be achieved using these same principles. For example, sportsmen and women have for years been using stretching techniques in order to prepare themselves for strenuous activity and to thus minimize the dangers of injury. Unfortunately, these often involve heroic stretching techniques, which sometimes in themselves cause damage to muscles and other soft tissues. Were the gentler Muscle Energy concepts utilized in an appropriate manner, this danger would be reduced.

Most of the methods which will be outlined in this chapter may be used selectively for particular regions of the body, or comprehensively to loosen most of the body, as desired. A few of the methods outlined are specific self-mobilization exercises which do not involve Muscle Energy, but rather utilize more direct release of tight structures.

> Care should be used in all of these not to involve force. The essence of self-treatment methods is that they should be safe and gentle. If any pain is ever associated with the preparation for, or the carrying out of any of the procedures described, then too much effort is being used, or the guidelines are not being followed accurately. Never do anything in self-treatment which causes more than transient, mild discomfort. In short, pain indicates a clear message to stop.

It is suggested that the procedures which are found to be successful should be repeated at least several times per week, and ideally every other day, if regained suppleness is to be maintained.

Variations on a theme of self-mobilization

A number of osteopathic and other physicians have, over the years, described different methods whereby they have been able to instruct and guide their patients in self-mobilization and treatment techniques. Over the next few pages of this chapter, a variety of these are presented. No indication can be given as to which will suit one person more than another. Try them all to see which feel more comfortable for you, which achieve greatest release of your particular tensions and tightnesses, and then incorporate these into a regular pattern, ideally to be used daily, or at least every other day.

Kirk's methods

Chester Kirk DO presented a sequence of exercises (and which I have modified slightly) in 1977 in the *Journal of the American Osteopathic Association*. All should be done in a relaxed manner, with a gentle degree of effort.

1. Sit in a straight chair, resting the palms of your hands on your thigh above your knees, fingers facing inwards.

   Allow the weight of your upper body to be supported by your arms by allowing your

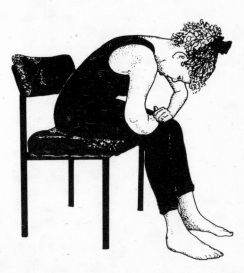

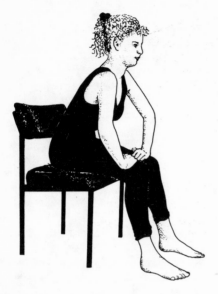

arm and hand, your body is taken into an upright position until a SLIGHT sense of strain or stretch is noted in your low back, and your hip or knee.

At this point, introduce a rhythmic pushing of the shoulders and trunk towards the midline, *always keeping your elbow straight*. The rhythm should be at a rate of about two per second, and this is best achieved by counting with each 'push' as follows: One-one, one-two; two-one, two-two; three-one, three-two; etc. until ten-two is reached.

At this point, stop for a few seconds and then repeat. The pushes against resistance (which is the tightness of the muscles of your low back preventing upright sitting) should be gentle, rapid and rhythmic, allowing a pulsating movement of the shoulders towards the midline at each count.

After about half a minute of these gentle repetitions, rest a moment and change position so that the other side can be stretched in the same manner.

3. Lie on your back on a carpeted floor,

elbows to bend outwards slightly as your head and chest come forwards, until a SLIGHT stretching sensation is felt in your low back. Hold for a count of five, breathing normally, and then push your upper body back to the starting position.

Repeat this five times.

It should be found that the lean forwards increases gradually with each repetition as your back muscles relax. Ideally your head should eventually get close to your knees.

2. Sit on the floor on one side of your buttocks, knees bent and both feet together on one side or the other. If sitting on your right buttock your feet would be on the left, with your right arm straight and extended to the right, your hand on the floor and some of the weight taken by that arm. Rest your left arm on your legs.

Pushing against the floor with your right

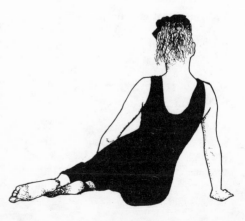

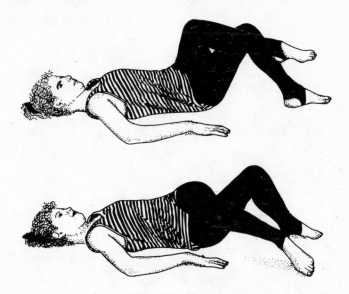

arms outstretched sideways, knees bent and your feet flat on the floor.

Raise one leg, still slightly bent at the knee, and cross it over your other leg allowing gravity to take that leg towards the floor until your foot touches it. This will pull your other knee towards the floor, placing a rotational twist on your low back. No resistance should be offered.

If any actual pain is felt as opposed to a feeling of stretching, stop immediately.

If your arm on the opposite side to which the twist is taking place wishes to rise from the floor, allow this to happen.

The foot which has gone across your body should then be gently lifted from the floor, from 3 to 6 inches, then allowed to perform a repetitive, bouncing action towards the floor and up again, about five times, springing the twisted segments of the body gently as it does so.

Return to the starting position and repeat on the other side of your body.

This effectively stretches your sacro-iliac, hip and shoulder regions.

4. Lie face upwards on the floor with your legs apart at a comfortable angle and your hands interlocked behind your neck.

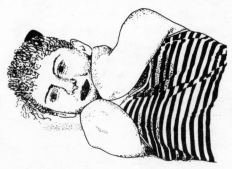

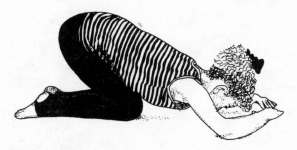

· Bring your elbows together and raise your head from the floor by a couple of inches.

Repetitively twist your trunk in opposite directions so that one elbow strikes the floor and then the other. Repeat so that this happens 5–10 times on each side.

This effectively stretches your mid-thoracic spine.

5. Imagine that you are going to roll a pea along the floor with your chin. This is the position to adopt for the next exercise.

Get onto your hands and knees with your thighs and arms perpendicular to the floor and your fingers pointing towards each other.

Bend your elbows to allow your head to drop towards your hands, but keep your head as upright as the position allows (i.e. not hanging downwards).

Take your chin as close to your hands as possible and slowly roll an invisible pea towards your knees with your chin.

Lift your head and shoulders and then take your chin towards your knees and slowly push an imaginary pea, with your chin, towards your hands. Then return to the starting position.

Repeat each variation five times.

Ideally the movements — beginning with the bending of your head towards your knees or hands, your chin rolling the pea forwards or backwards and the return to the raised head position — should all be accomplished with your breath exhaled.

Thus, the movement starts as your breath is being exhaled. The next breath is not taken until assuming the position on all fours with your head and shoulders away from the floor.

If a rotational stretch is needed in your upper back, then a modification of the above can be achieved by introducing a turn of the head through each of the positions described. In this case one could imagine that a pea was being rolled forwards or backwards by one or other ear.

Ideally, several, but not more than five of each of the variations should be performed.

6. Kirk suggests a modified yoga position to stretch the lower back and trunk effectively.

Sit on the floor with your legs out-stretched. Cross your left leg over your right leg at the knees. Cross your right arm over your legs and place your right hand between your crossed knees. This tends to lock the position of your legs.

Your left hand is then taken behind your body and placed on the floor 6–8 inches behind your buttocks with your fingers pointing backwards. This twist should be done to the limit available involving a full but painless rotation of your shoulders and trunk to the left.

Your head should also then be turned as far to the left as possible, looking over your shoulder.

Stay in this position whilst you take a series of slow breaths in and out.

At the end of this time, try to increase slightly the range of rotation before return-

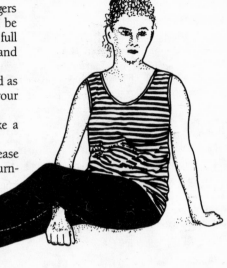

ing to the upright, untwisted position and before repeating the whole procedure on the other side. In other words, alter and reverse all positions described above.

No pain should be felt, but a feeling of a good deal of stretch is desirable.

Resistive duction methods

The method of repetitive pushing against a resistance as used in exercise 2. above, was first described by the osteopathic physician

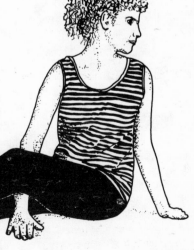

T.J. Ruddy in the 1960s. He called this method Osteopathic Rhythmic Resistive Duction Therapy. This simple method has been found to be very useful since it effectively accomplishes a number of changes simultaneously, involving nerve impulses, fluid exchange, oxygen exchange, drainage of breakdown products, reduction of contraction etc. The term 'pulsed muscle energy' is one I now use to describe Ruddy's safe and effective method, which depends entirely for its effectiveness on the 'pulsed' efforts being very light indeed, *with no 'wobble' or 'bounce' produced, just the barest activation of the muscles involved.*

An example of this method in terms of self-mobilization is the following:

Sit at a table, rest a hand on it, tilt your head forwards and rest your hand against your forehead.

Use a rhythm of pressure by your head (as though taking it forwards into flexion) against the resistance of your hand of one-one, one-two; two-one, two-two; three-one, etc. until ten-two is reached.

This will relax your muscles of the region, especially those involved in flexion.

Variations may be used for all positions of movement of your head or any other part of your body.

If pain is felt, push less hard.

This method may be employed against the fixed resistance, of one's own or a friend's hands, just as in the Muscle Energy methods described in earlier chapters. Use the positions outlined in the Muscle Energy chapters, for the various regions of the body, in order to create a starting position for Resistive Duction exercises, whenever a feeling of tightness or restriction is noted.

The key to the successful use of it is to apply 20 painless contractions, against resistance, in 10 seconds. This can be repeated several times or until tenderness and restriction ease.

Additional self-mobilization methods

A series of additional self-mobilization methods derived from osteopathic sources are given below. Some of these are modifications of the work of Lawrence Jones DO, the developer of Strain/counterstrain, who also advocated self-treatment wherever possible and desirable.

General spinal stretching

1. Lie face upwards on a carpeted floor, a pillow under your head.

Flex your knees so that your feet, which should be together, are flat on the floor.

Keep your shoulders in contact with the floor, a situation which is aided by having your arms stretched sideways, palms upwards.

Allow both your knees to fall to the right as far as possible without pain. This imposes a twist on your lower and middle back muscles.

Allow the weight of your legs to create the effort, and the inertia of the rest of your body to act as counter-force to this isometric effort. Your shoulders and feet should be flat on the floor all the while.

Breathe deeply and slowly for about 30 seconds, then take a deep breath held for a further 15-20 seconds.

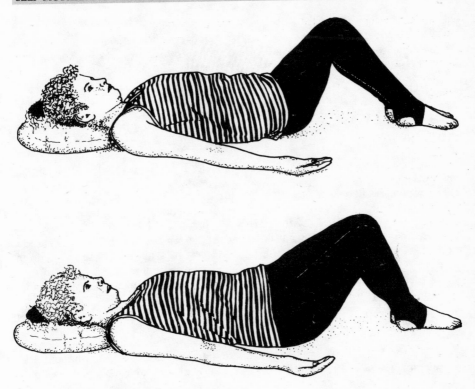

On release of the breath allow your legs to fall further towards the floor. Stay in this position for another 15–20 seconds.

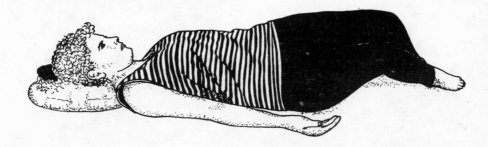

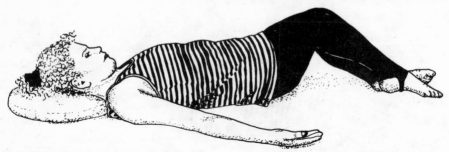

2. Bring your knees back to the midline and repeat on the left.

3. Lie flat on the floor legs outstretched, arms by your side.

Keeping your outstretched legs together, take them to one side or the other as far as is possible from the midline and rest them there.

Take your head and shoulders slowly in the same direction as far as is comfortably possible and rest in this position. A full sidebend will have been achieved.

You should now be lying in a rough C-shape. Simply maintain this sidebent posture for a period of 30 seconds, during which you should breathe deeply, then hold your breath for a further 15-20 seconds.

On exhalation of this breath, try to take your legs and your upper body slightly further to the side to increase the stretch.

Hold this for a further 15-20 seconds.

A variation of this position would be, during the whole of the procedure, to put your arm on the side to which you are bending, extended towards your feet, whilst the other was extended above your head.

4. Come back to the midline and perform the same procedure on the other side.

5. Lie on one side or the other, pillow under your head.

Keeping your legs together, one resting on the other, bend your knees and curl up into a bent position so that your back is as rounded as possible. Try to bring your nose as close to your knees as possible without any pain.

Ensure that your neck or head is supported by a cushion all the time.

Breathe deeply, then relax for 30 seconds. This is equivalent to approximately three cycles of complete inhalation and exha-

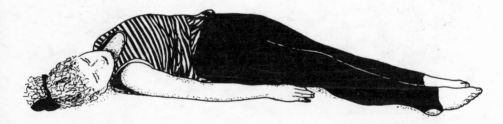

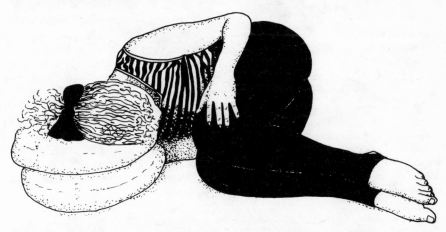

lation if slowly performed. Then take a deep breath and hold it for 15–20 seconds.

On exhalation try to curl a little further, and stay in this position for another 15–20 seconds.

6. Return to the straight position and, keeping your legs together one on the other, and backwards or folded on your chest during this, but your neck and head should always be supported.

Hold this position for 30 seconds whilst breathing deeply and slowly. Then hold your breath for a further 15–20 seconds and, on exhalation, try to stretch a little further.

Hold this for a further 15–20 seconds.

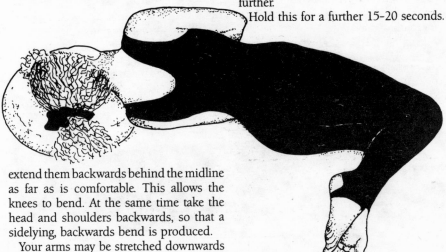

extend them backwards behind the midline as far as is comfortable. This allows the knees to bend. At the same time take the head and shoulders backwards, so that a sidelying, backwards bend is produced.

Your arms may be stretched downwards

Remember that no pain should ever be experienced during or after the positions described. If it is, then you are forcing yourself beyond a comfortable stretch, which is all that is being asked.

This series of positions, all performed in a manner which avoids the force of gravity being superimposed, allows multiple releases of tight structures using a combin-ation of reciprocal inhibition and post isometric relaxation. A good deal of free-dom of movement should be felt thereafter, especially after this has been done on a number of occasions, ideally every other day.

After the first few such sessions it is normal to expect a degree of generalized muscle ache and stiffness as though strenuous exercise had been undertaken. This is quite normal and indicates nothing more than that the regions stretched were in need of this.

Additional methods of stretching and loosening particular regions

For thigh and hip muscles

1. Lie on the floor or a bed. Create an isometric contraction by placing one foot on top of the other.

Keeping both knees straight, try to pull upwards towards the body with your lower foot and leg, whilst with your upper foot and leg you try to push away from your body. If your leg muscles as a whole are allowed to join in this struggle of opposing forces, rather than just the feet, a better result will be achieved.

Maintain the contractions, using about 30 per cent of the strength available, for 10 seconds or so, and then release.

Immediately after release, push the leg which was pulling upwards, away from the body, all the way from the hip, as though

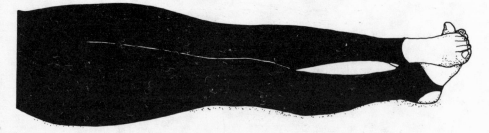

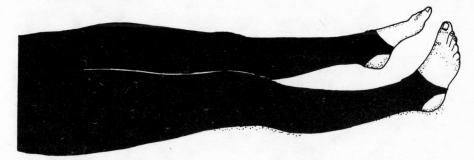

you were trying to reach something distant from you with your heel. Ensure that your low back stays flat during this stretch. Hold this position for 10 seconds and then relax. Repeat the isometric contraction with your other foot on top, and then after release stretch your lower leg away from your hips as far as possible for 10 seconds.

For lower back and back of thigh

1. Lie face upwards, cushion under your head. Keep one leg straight. Bend the other at the hip and knee. Place your hands under your knee to grasp your lower thigh and pull this leg to your chest as close as is comfortable. Hold this position and your breath for 7-10 seconds. As you release

your breath pull your leg a little closer to your chest. Ensure that your other leg remains straight during all this.

Repeat with the other leg.

2. Lying on your back, no cushion. Bend both legs at the hip and knee. With legs apart and a hand on each knee, pull your legs towards their respective shoulders.

When the position closest to your shoulders is reached, hold this and your breath for 10 seconds. As your breath is released pull your knees a little closer to your shoulders, not your chest, and hold again for 10 seconds as another breath is held. (See illustration overleaf.)

Repeat until no further gain is achieved in approximation of knees to shoulders.

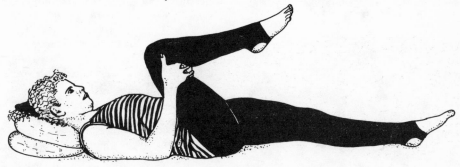

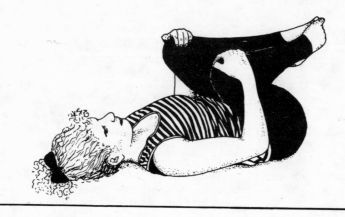

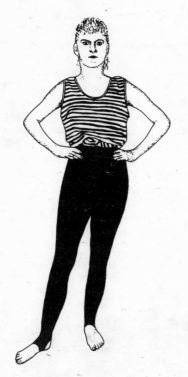

To stretch, by means of repetitive exercise, a tight iliotibial band (tensor fascia lata)

This structure runs from above the hip joint to below the knee, on the outside of the leg. If it is tight, it can contribute to recurrent low back pain, recurrent sacro-iliac problems and also to knee and hip dysfunction.

A number of Muscle Energy methods are outlined in Chapter 4 which can assist in normalization, as can the following exercises:

1. To stretch the right Iliotibial Band
Stand with the heel of your right foot in the hollow of your left foot so that your foot faces away from the midline by about 25°.

Advance your right foot half a step forwards and slightly outwards and place your body weight on to your right leg. With your right leg thus braced at your knee, your upper leg should have been effectively rotated outwards in relation to your body, placing strain on the fibres of the iliotibial band.

Keeping your hips level, move your pelvis to the right, and in doing so allow the heel of your left foot to rise slightly as your left knee bends to accommodate this movement.

Hold this position for a few seconds and then move your pelvis back to the midline before repeating the stretch of the tight fibres. Do this 10-20 times at least three times daily.

Ensure that when your pelvis is translated to the right that it does not tilt. Your right shoulder would drop, and this would negate the benefits.

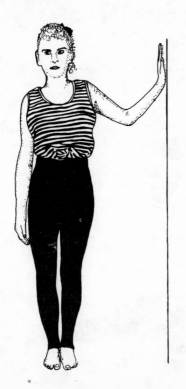

Repeat on your other leg if indicated.

2. Stand an arm's length from a wall, the side to be stretched closer to the wall. If the left side is to be stretched, stand with your left side closer to the wall, your left arm outstretched and your palm upwards against the wall. Allow your outstretched arm to bend, thus bringing your body closer to the wall and placing a stretch on the outside of your left leg.

This is only effective if your trunk remains upright and your pelvis remains parallel with the floor, and is not allowed to dip towards the wall as the exercise is performed.

Hold this for several seconds and then return to an upright position before repeating.

Repeat 10-20 times two or three times daily instead of exercise 1. above or alternating with it.

Repeat on your other leg if necessary.

To stretch the muscles and soft tissues on the front and outside of the thigh, including the iliotibial band

Adopt the starting position as used in sprinting. Place one foot in front of your body, flat and facing forwards. The foot of your leg which extends behind your trunk, the leg being treated, is placed so that weight is taken on the ball of your foot, flexing it. This foot should be rotated to face inwards.

In this position tension should be felt on the front/outer aspect of your upper leg.

By repetitively flexing your front knee, additional stretch is placed on these fibres, especially if the knee on your extended leg is kept from bending.

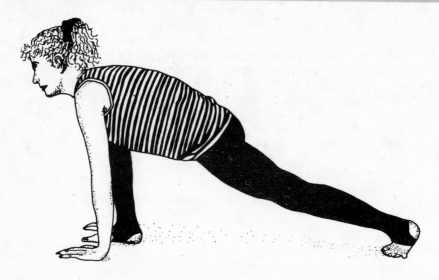

Repeat this knee flexing to stretch the tight fibres 20–30 times.

To mobilize the sacro-iliac joint

Lie on the unaffected side with the lower leg straight. Allow the knee of the upper leg, which is flexed at hip and knee, to rest on the floor, thus stabilizing the pelvis.

Place the palm of the upper hand on the prominent front portion of the pelvic bone so that the palm faces downwards to the floor.

Repetitively and rhythmically 'spring' this bone in a direction roughly towards the lower ribs on the other side, without any great force, for about 20 seconds.

The repetitive downward (to the floor) and headward direction of the springing action causes a gentle gapping at the back of the pelvis, where the sacro-iliac joint is found.

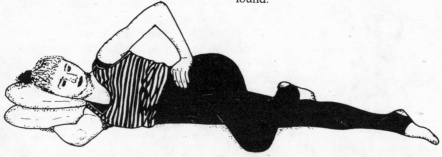

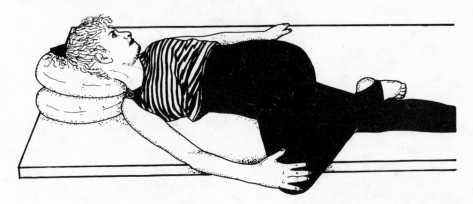

To mobilize the lumbar spine

Lie on the side close to the edge of a bed or table.

The lower leg is outstretched while the upper leg is flexed at hip and knee, so the foot rests behind the outstretched leg. For the lower lumbar spine the toes rest below the knee.

The upper hand is taken behind the body to grasp the edge of the table/bed. Taking the upper body into rotation, face upwards, rest the lower hand on the flexed knee, which should be over the edge of the table/bed.

There now exists a good degree of torsion between the upper and lower body. No pain should be felt.

Initially, there should be a deep inhalation and at the same time a turning of the head to its maximum extent away from the edge of the bed, over which the flexed knee is lying. At the same time, the hand resting on that knee exerts mild downward (to the floor) pressure to create an increase in the rotation.

This is held for 10 seconds. Then the pressure downwards, the turning away of the head, and the breath are all released simultaneously.

This may be repeated once or twice more.

Then the head is again turned away from the bed. The hand on the knee then exerts a rhythmic downwards springing motion at a rate of roughly once or twice per second, for no more than a minute.

For the upper lumbar spine, exactly the same position and procedure is required, except that the foot of the upper leg rests above the knee of the lower leg, while the lower leg is very slightly flexed at the knee. Whichever procedure is performed this should also be done lying on the other side, afterwards, which involves all the low back muscles on both sides.

To mobilize the thoracic spine

Kneel on a carpeted floor so that the weight is taken on the flexed knees and elbows. The thighs should be at right angles to the floor.

For the upper thoracic spine have the elbows level with the ears. Breathe in deeply and arch the back as far as is possible,

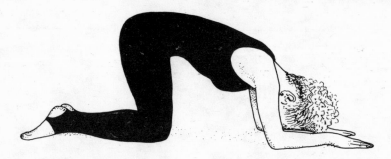

allowing the head to drop to the floor. This rounds the thoracic spine.

Try to imagine as this is being done that the navel is being pulled upwards to meet the spine, thus effectively increasing the degree of arching.

The breath and the position should be held for 5 seconds or so and then released at the same time as lowering the thoracic spine towards the floor and raising the head.

This effectively flattens and depresses the thoracic spine. Hold this position for 5 seconds before inhaling and arching again. Repeat five or six times in each direction.

In order to localize the effect at the junction of the lumbar and thoracic spine,

a most important transition area where the spinal curves change direction, the hands rather than the elbows should be used for support.

All other aspects of the procedure remain the same.

To localize mobilization of the upper thoracic spine and ribs

Sit on the edge of a table, knees apart with head bowed forwards.

Allow one arm to hang between the legs and the other down the outside one of the legs. If the arm between the legs was the left one then the other arm would hang by the outer side of the right leg.

Make sure the shoulder blades are

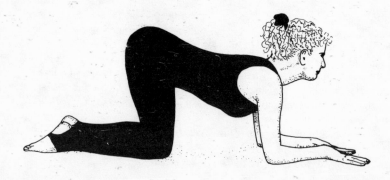

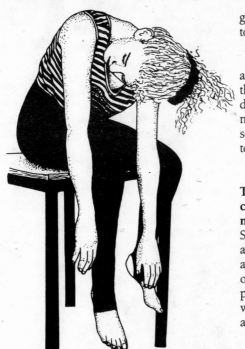

gravity to stretch the head and the arms towards the floor.

Repeat once or twice more.

Keeping this position, with only gravity acting on the arms and the head turned to the same side as above, breathe slowly and deeply; try to 'breathe into' the tight areas noted in the upper back. This produces a separation of the ribs in this area and helps to mobilize the region further.

Repeat all the above on the other side.

To assist in mobilization of the cervicothoracic junction area, where the neck meets the trunk

Sit on the edge of a bed or table. Stretch the arms sideways with fingers widely spread, and rotate the arms at the shoulder, in opposite directions, so that one is turned palm backwards and the other palm upwards or forwards. Ensure that the arms are actually stretched out straight.

relaxed, and are not held in tension. The head should be turned to the right.

Take a deep breath and at the same time as turning the head to its maximum degree of rotation to the right, (i.e. in this example), stretch the left arm downwards towards the floor.

Hold the stretch and the breath for 10 seconds, and on release relax in that position for a further 10 seconds, allowing

Turn the head towards the side on which the hand is turned backwards, with the thumb facing the floor.

After 3-5 seconds rotate the arms in opposite directions and simultaneously turn the head to the other side on which the thumb now faces the floor.

Ensure that the shoulders are not hunched but are as relaxed as possible. Try to synchronize the movement of the head and arms with a deep breath in, sighing the breath out slowly as the position is held. As the next breath is taken in, rotate the arms and turn the head.

Repeat 10 times.

For general mobilization of the cervical spine see the Muscle Energy methods described at the beginning of Chapter 4, as well as the various Muscle Energy methods for neck structures in that chapter.

For a general stretch of the upper thoracic/lower cervical (neck) muscles

Lie face down with the elbows together resting just fowards of a line running from shoulder to shoulder. This elevates the upper back and if the head is allowed to hang free imposes a stretch on the junction area of neck and trunk.

With the head hanging thus in the mid-line, breathe in and raise the head an inch or so whilst holding the breath for 7-10 seconds. On exhalation, allow the head to

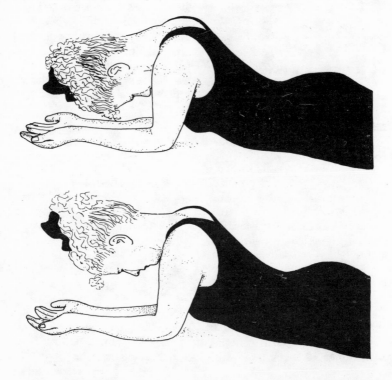

hang freely for a further 10 seconds before repeating once or twice more.

Variations can include having the head turned slightly one way or the other and performing the same isometric contraction.

A number of simple exercises exist for retraining muscles controlling the jaw which have become disturbed

Facing a mirror, place toothpicks between the midline upper and lower teeth. Slowly open and close the mouth, ensuring that the toothpicks remain one above the other all the time.

As they deviate from this line, bring them together again in this manner, thus training them to be symmetrically balanced.

The muscle (usually the pterygoid) which is tight will have to slacken off and its antagonist will have to tighten, to bring about harmonious and symmetrical motion. This midline exercise should be done many times daily by individuals with **temperomandibular joint (TMJ) problems**.

A further exercise involves curling the tongue upwards so that the tip touches the roof of the mouth as far back as possible.

Keeping this in place, open and close the mouth slowly. This tongue position prevents the jaw from coming forwards. Perform this many times daily if there is TMJ dysfunction.

To help retrain neck and shoulder muscles which may be being used inappropriately in breathing

Sit in an upright chair which has arms, resting your elbows on these. Push

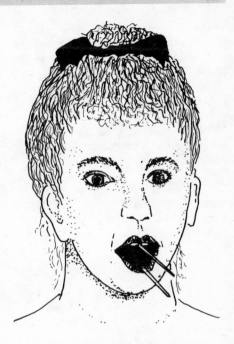

Exercise using toothpicks between midline upper and lower teeth to retrain jaw muscles — the idea is to keep the toothpicks aligned whilst slowly opening and closing the mouth

moderately firmly downwards with the elbows while taking a series of slow deep breaths (counting 3 or 4 as you inhale and 4 or 5 as you slowly exhale). The downward elbow pressure prevents the shoulders from being raised and forces a more correct use of many associate respiratory muscles. This may feel odd at first, but repeat the breathing cycle 10 to 15 times, 3 or 4 times daily, until the correct muscles are retrained.

This type of problem is common in people with asthma, bronchial disorders and those with a tendency to hyperventilate. This method should be accompanied by stretching of muscles such as the scalenes, trapezius, levator scapulae and sternocleidomastoid (see Chapter 4) all of which may shorten when this form of inappropriate breathing is apparent.

Always remember to sit quietly for a few minutes after deep breathing in case of transient dizziness.

These examples of general and specific stretching techniques and mobilization methods do not of course cover every area of the body. They should permit a good deal of increased freedom of movement in the spinal regions and assist in the loosening of many of the tight tissues which contribute towards postural and general dysfunction.

A good book on Yoga, or better still attending a class, will assist in expanding on the concepts outlined in this chapter.

Remember that at no time when any of these exercises/manoeuvres are being performed should actual pain be felt. Discomfort afterwards, as experienced after vigorous exercise is acceptable, but not pain.

7

Strain and counterstrain techniques

A well-known osteopathic physician in the USA, Lawrence Jones DO, was confronted some years ago by a particularly difficult patient who was in such pain that even getting him onto the treatment table was a major undertaking.

Despite using all his considerable skills Jones was seldom able to relieve the patient more than slightly and he came to dread the repetitive visits. On one occasion the procedure of getting the patient into a relatively painless position on the table took so long that most of the scheduled appointment time had been used up by the time this was actually achieved. Since other patients were by now waiting for his attention elsewhere, Jones left the patient resting in what was for him a tolerably comfortable posture, but which was in fact a slight exaggeration of the distorted position in which the stooped and agonised patient usually stood. Returning after twenty minutes or so Jones asked how the patient was and was surprised to hear a cheerful response of 'fine'. Since there was no time to treat the man, Jones assisted him from the table only to discover to his (and the patient's) amazement, that he was now pain-free, and able to stand erect.

Jones had stumbled on a method for obliging the body to spontaneously release spasm, and it led him to research deeply into this phenomenon and to develop a system which has come to be known as Strain/counterstrain technique.

This system has several strands, one of which is the recognition of what should be obvious. When the body is distorted because of muscular spasm, any attempt to try to straighten it meets with the response of increased pain, and thus more spasm. Jones discovered that by taking the entire body, or specific area, further in the direction of distortion, by actually exaggerating it, something rather amazing could occur. If this exaggeration was precisely as it should be (see below) the spasm released, not immediately, but after a short while.

In his research, Jones discovered something else as well. Most joint strains have associated with them localized areas of marked tenderness. These can be used to tell the patient and the operator (practitioner etc.) in which direction the joint or area wants to go. If a tender point, as Jones called it, was located, it should be pressed lightly while the strained or injured joint is taken in various directions. In some directions, the pain felt in the 'tender' point will be found to increase, while in other directions it will decrease or vanish altogether.

When the precise position of maximum ease is found for the joint, in which the tenderness in the tender point vanishes or markedly reduces, nothing else needs to be done, except to stay still in that position, for at least a minute and a half (90 seconds). This is the time it takes for the affected muscles' neurological reporting stations, (muscle spindles and other minute structures which constantly send the central nervous system a series of integrated messages as to the status of the muscles and tendons in which they lie and without which co-ordinated movement is impossible), to start sending coherent messages to the central nervous system, obliging it to shut off the spasm and over-contraction. This is what produced the relief from pain and spasm when the over-exaggeration of the distorted body position was engineered in Jones' first, unintentional, strain/counterstrain patient.

We now have two strong guides as to how to deal with joint dysfunction or muscle strain in which muscular spasm or contraction is holding an area in an unnatural manner, preventing normal use and function.

While the position is maintained for 90 seconds, so also is the pressure contact on the tender point, since it is important that no deviation from the exact position of ease occurs during these 90 seconds. If it did the tender point would begin to palpate as sensitive.

The tender point thus becomes our personal information source as it indicates whether or not we are in the right position. This 'functional' technique has, along with Muscle Energy Technique, revolutionized manipulative work, since it allows the physiological response of the body to achieve what was previously achieved only

by great effort on the part of the osteopath or chiropractor. The methods are less stressful to the practitioner, far more pleasant for the patient, take less time and in terms of self-treatment they offer another safe method for dealing with strains and sprains.

Another of Jones' discoveries was that the position of ease, in which the tender point feels less sensitive or in which there is pain-free exaggeration of distortion, are in fact usually duplications of the position in which the original strain or injury occurred.

For example, if someone is standing on a ladder and painting a ceiling and they subsequently develop a pain in the low neck or shoulder, it is probable that some strain occurred whilst in a position where the arm was extended and the neck was tilted back. It is in some variation of this position that either the pain itself would feel considerably reduced, or the pain noted in a tender point being contacted by a probing finger would reduce (in such a strain the tender point would be located around the base of the neck).

We are all familiar with the stooped position adopted by anyone with 'lumbago'. Try to force them to stand erect and the screams would soon stop the effort. Ask the stooped individual to bend further however, and often this is easily and painlessly achieved. Ask this individual if they recall how it started, and often you will be told that they were bending, lifting or carrying something awkward when a pain was felt, and they have been stuck in this way ever since.

The fascinating final piece of Jones' jigsaw puzzle is discovered when it is reported that the tender point in a condition which resulted from bending forwards is not to be found in the region of the pain which they feel in their back, but rather on the front of the body, in the abdominal muscles. The tender point for the injured low neck was found on the back of the body near the spine, when the injury occurred with the individual stretching up and bending backwards. In the same way the tender point for a forward-bending strain can be found on the front surface of the body.

If a strain occurs in a twisted or sidebent position then there would also be a more lateral location of the tender point, than if the strain had occurred in simply bending forwards or backwards.

How can we use this knowledge in self-treatment?

If we know how a strain took place, we can use that knowledge to help us to locate the tender point, which can subsequently be used as a guide to help find the position of maximum ease, the position of release. If we do not know in what position the strain took place we may have to experiment and search in order to find either a position of maximum ease in terms of an existing pain or of a tender point which is found on palpation, and which we can use as our guide to find a position of release.

Fortunately, much of this detective work is not always necessary, for Jones has, with great care, charted the major sites of tender points in relation to a host of different joint strains. Guidance will be given as to some of these.

The key to successful employment of this system lies in the use of either the pain itself or the tender point as guides to the best position, in terms of ease from discomfort. A general direction can be given for most joints as to how to position them in order to find the position of ease. A degree of 'fine tuning' is often necessary though, to find the precise position where the maximum degree of ease is felt, as indicated by the reduced degree of tenderness in the point.

After this, all that is required is maintenance of the position of ease for 90 seconds and a constant contact with the tender point to ensure that no deviation from this position occurs. Follow this by slow and careful use of the whole body or specific area until full recovery is achieved. In self-treatment, using this method, the use of the tender point as guide is suggested as the most accurate way of identifying the position of ease.

The following are a number of the most common of Jones' tender point sites relating to spinal strains.

In some but not all of the examples given below, great detail will be gone into as to the possible variations in position. In others only an outline is given. It is suggested that you carefully read and follow the detailed examples, then use the same principles as in the outlined examples.

Neck strain (Forward bending):

Tender points for strain of the 1st cervical vertebra, if strained in forwards bending, may be found between the angle of the jaw and the mastoid process behind the ear (a), or alternatively there may be one just in front of the angle of the jaw (b).

You should be lying on a bed or the floor

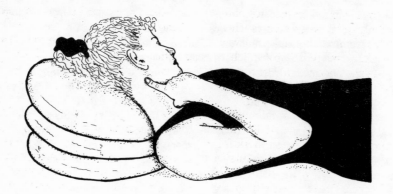

Shows C1 flexion strain. With a finger contacting tender point — flex neck and rotate away from pain side until tenderness abates — hold for 90 seconds

with a cushion under the head to introduce forward bending of the head.

Having located the tender point, apply pressure to it sufficient to produce tenderness locally.

The position of ease for (a) is usually found by flexing the neck, that is bending it forwards gently, turning it away from the side of the painful point and perhaps also bending it a little to the side.

It may be necessary to experiment with more or less bending forwards, more or less rotation away from the side of pain, and more or less sidebending (taking the ear towards the shoulder). Do this until the most relaxed position is found, as indicated by the tender point being less tender or not tender at all any more.

For (b) it is also necessary to flex the neck and to rotate it away from the side of pain, but its fine tuning usually involves a side-

bend towards the painful side.

In either (a) or (b), when the ideal position is found in which the most ease from the tenderness in the point is felt, stay in that position, maintain finger contact on the point and do nothing else for at least 90 seconds.

Release the pressure and slowly return the neck to its neutral position. In rare instances in type (a) it is found that rotation and sidebending *towards* the side of pain is the only way to take out the tenderness. This highlights the fact that although guidelines can be given, as they are throughout this chapter, individual elements enter into strains which means that we have to seek out the exact position of ease by trial and error, if the guidelines do not produce the correct position.

The guidelines given are the most usual ones, in any given type of spinal joint strain, for finding the position of ease. They are not, however, infallibly correct.

For strains which occurred in bending forwards and which are affecting the 2nd to the 6th cervical vertebrae inclusive, the tender points are located on the tips of the corresponding transverse processes. These are the bones which protrude sideways from the vertebrae and the tips of which, in the cervical region, are felt in a line running down the side of the neck, roughly in line with the ear.

Lying on the floor with a cushion under the head, the positions of ease for these points are found by flexing the neck forwards, rotating it away from the painful side and sometimes, especially in the region of C5 and C6, sidebending away from the painful side as well.

An idiosyncratic vertebra in this section is C4 in which, instead of bending the head forwards (flexing), it is taken backwards

Shows C5/6 flexion strain. With contact on tender point — flex neck and rotate away from pain side until tenderness abates — hold for 90 seconds

slightly, into extension, before rotating away from the pain.

This is achieved by placing the cushion under the upper back, thus allowing the head and neck to slightly extend over it.

Palpate the tender point, place the head into flexion (or if C4 is involved into extension), gently rotate and, if indicated, sidebend until the tenderness vanishes.

Stay in that position for 90 seconds.

In forward-bending strains affecting the 7th cervical (the last of the neck vertebrae), the tender point is usually found on the upper surface of the collarbone (clavicle), near its junction with the breastbone (sternum). Flex the head and rotate away from the pain, and, usually, sidebend towards it, to find the position of maximum ease. This is best accomplished lying face upwards on the floor or a bed, with a cushion under the neck or head.

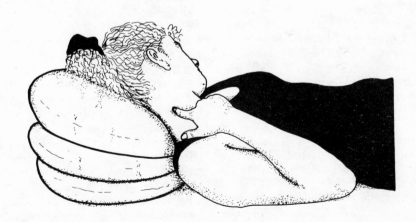

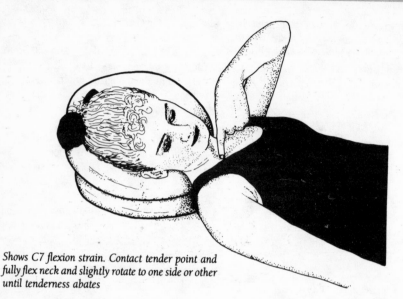

Shows C7 flexion strain. Contact tender point and fully flex neck and slightly rotate to one side or other until tenderness abates

Neck Strain (Backward bending):

The treatment of extension strains (backward bending) usually involves taking the area into extension.

This is best achieved in the neck region, in self-treatment, by lying on the side, with the painful side uppermost.

A variation is possible in which by lying face upwards near the edge of the bed the head may be allowed to extend over the edge, placing the neck into extension.

The sidelying posture is that recommended for self-use.

Extension strain of the 1st cervical vertebra produces tender points in (a) the muscles at the base of the skull or (b) just to the side of the prominence on the skull which lies just above the occiput (the inion).

For (a), locate the tender point and extend the head and rotate it towards the side of the pain. Fine tuning is achieved by increasing the degree of extension, not of the neck itself, but of the head on the neck (i.e. tilt the head slightly backwards on the neck).

For (b) the opposite is required, so that maximum flexion is applied to the neck, thus placing the chin on the upper chest or lower throat. No rotation is usually needed for (b) as the pain felt to the side of the inion, on pressure of the tender point, will usually vanish as the head is taken forwards.

Hold appropriate position for (a) or (b) for 90 seconds then slowly release.

Extension strains of 2nd cervical to 7th cervical inclusive produce tender points close to the spine itself, in the groove lying

Shows C1 extension strain. Contact tender point and extend (bend backwards) neck and rotate towards pain side (plus sometimes side-bending) until tenderness abates

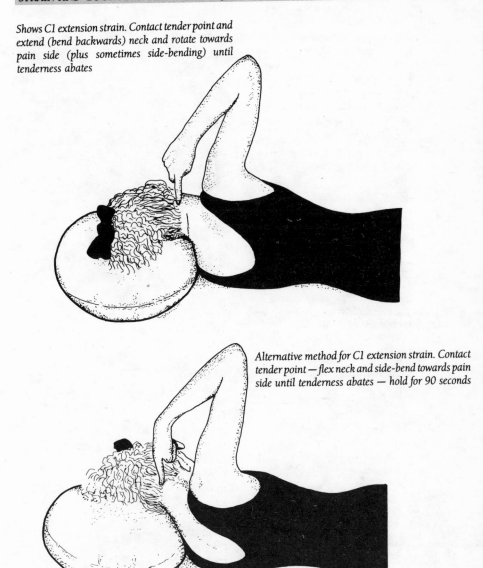

Alternative method for C1 extension strain. Contact tender point — flex neck and side-bend towards pain side until tenderness abates — hold for 90 seconds

alongside the prominent bones on the midline (the spinous processes).

Lie on the side, with the painful side uppermost and the head on a cushion, so that it is kept in the midline and is not allowed to tilt sideways. Take the head and neck backwards and rotate towards the painful side. If fine tuning is not being successful in easing the tenderness introduce sidebending as well, until maximum ease is noted in the tender point.

Hold for 90 seconds.

The exception to this is the 3rd cervical which instead of being taken backwards should be taken into flexion, in most instances.

There are other variations in dealing with neck strains, but these examples are the simplest and safest and will allow most people to relieve themselves of pain from recent strain, including whiplash type injuries, which took place in extension.

Note: It is suggested that if by following the guidelines given in this section it is not possible to positionally ease the tender point pain, try variations until you find the right position.

The body will always tell you when you are in the correct position of ease. Always position areas slowly and in a controlled manner, never quickly and never, never to produce increased pain of any sort. This is essentially the most gentle of methods and should under no circumstances involve pain during positioning or holding of the position adopted for ease, apart from the initial tenderness felt in the 'tender' point. If any other pain is noted stop immediately, and consult a trained osteopath.

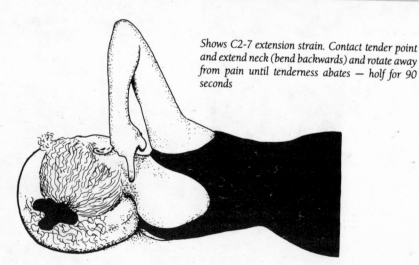

Shows C2-7 extension strain. Contact tender point and extend neck (bend backwards) and rotate away from pain until tenderness abates — holf for 90 seconds

Flexion strains of the thoracic spine

The treatment of flexion strains in the thoracic region of the spine involves positioning the body in a curled up or flexed position.

Lie on the back with the knees bent up, and a cushion under the head, or adopt a curled up, side-lying position. The tender points for 1st thoracic vertebral strain which occurred in flexion (forward bending), lie in the hollow above the sternum (breast bone).

Fine tuning involves taking the head into full forward bending with slight rotation to one side or the other until the tenderness in the point is much reduced or nonexistent. This is held for 90 seconds.

Flexion strains of the 2nd to 6th thoracic vertebrae produce tender points on the sternum itself, roughly half an inch apart.

Treatment position for these is as for the 1st thoracic, involving more or less flexion, directing the head towards one or other foot, introducing in this way a degree of sidebending/rotation.

The lower the problem, the more essential it is to ensure overall flexion by bringing the knees well up towards the chest as the neck and upper back flexion/sidebending is introduced.

The tender point for 7th thoracic forward bending strain is found either just below or slightly to the side of the small prominence at the base of the sternum, the xyphoid process.

Treatment position is as for the 1st to 6th thoracic as above.

It is usually also possible to produce the desired degree of flexion in the supine (face upwards) position by prodigious use of cushions to build up and support the desired curve of the back.

A cushion under the buttocks, flexed knees and several cushions under the neck/head/upper back can produce the

First thoracic glexion strain

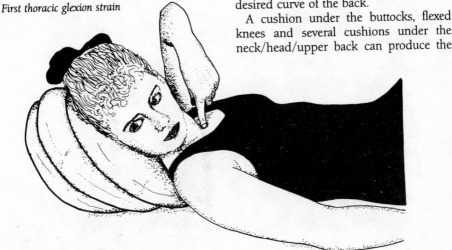

desired position, although it can be time consuming finding the precise position of ease.

Self-treatment in the sidelying position should be attempted first, as this reduces the need for cushions.

Treatment of forward bending strains of the 8th to 12th thoracic vertebrae involves similar positioning; a cushion under the buttocks, flexed knees supported on a low stool or the seat of a chair, the head and upper back supported by cushions etc.

The knees are taken more to one side or the other as they are flexed upwards, in order to find the precise point of ease of tenderness in the points.

A degree of sidebending to, or away from, the side of pain may also be introduced in fine tuning, with the ankles crossed, or not, as a further refinement.

12th thoracic flexion strain. Contact tender point — introduce flexion by supporting upper and lower parts of body together with side-bending until tenderness abates — hold for 90 seconds

Treatment of the 12th thoracic (see below for its location) requires more sidebending than the other spinal strains, indeed the necessary degree of flexion also usually increases for the lower points.

The positions of the tender points for lower thoracic flexion strains are as follows:

The 10th thoracic is about half an inch below the navel. The 8th and 9th are 3 inches and 1 inch respectively above the 10th.

The 11th thoracic is about an inch and a half below the 10th, and the 12th is near the bony prominence at the front of the pelvic bone, the anterior superior spine of the iliac crest.

Extension strains of the thoracic spine

Just as the tender points for extension (backward-bending) strains of the neck region were found near the spine, so are the extension strain points in the thoracic spine.

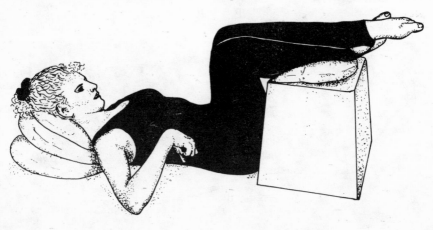

1st-4th thoracic extension strain

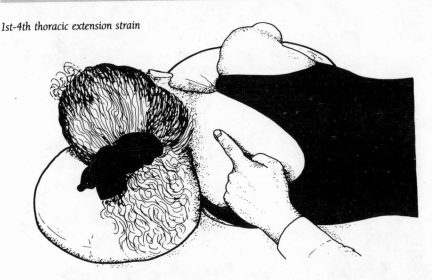

The 1st thoracic vertebral extension strain tender point is found near the spinous process, close to the midline.

The lower the strain in the thoracic spine the more to the side the tender point is located, with 12th thoracic extension strain tender points being located near the tip of the transverse process, the part of the spine that protrudes sideways and which in this region articulates with the ribs. It is very difficult, if not impossible, to maintain a pressure contact on a tender point in this region when self-treatment is being performed. Some degree of assistance is therefore necessary for this function, as well as to assist in the supply of cushions for support in the positioning stage of the treatment.

Treatment of extension strains involves backwards bending.

The suggested position is lying on the affected side.

A pillow should be used to support the upper arm (place this between the arms) so that no twisting of the upper body occurs in this position.

For 1st to 4th thoracic extension strains, lie on the side, with the arm positioned level with shoulders. Backward bending of the head/neck produces extension of the thoracic spine.

This and a degree of rotation and side-bending of the head (usually away from the affected side) is used for fine tuning. Use cushions to support the final position, with the assistance of someone to supply and position these, as the tender point is monitored for lessening sensitivity.

Hold for 90 seconds once the position of maximum ease is achieved.

For 5th to 8th thoracic extension strains, sidelying is also suggested, with the arms above head level and supported, as above, to

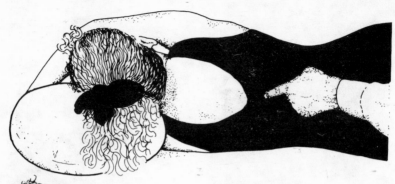

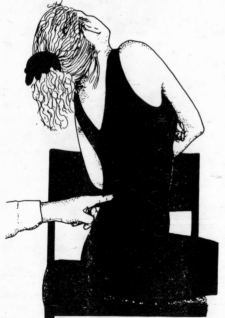

5th-8th thoracic extension strain. Backward bending of head/neck and slight rotation and/or side-bending until tenderness abates — hold for 90 seconds

avoid twisting of the upper body.

For 9th to 12th thoracic extension strains, sit with arms folded, then bend slightly backwards to produce extension. Experiment with a degree of rotation and side-bending towards or away from the side of the tender point, in order to find the position of maximum ease in the tender point.

Or, lie face down with a pillow under the chest to permit backwards bending, and a cushion under the hip on the side of the tender point. Cushions of various thicknesses need to be tried until maximum ease is felt in the tender point.

Assistance is obviously required for the positioning as well as for the monitoring of the tender point.

9th-12th thoracic extension strain. Fold arms and lean back until tenderness abates — hold for 90 seconds
Note: assistance is required in this position to maintain contact on tender point — self treatment is not possible

Flexion strains of the lumbar spine

The positioning for these strains is similar to that used for thoracic flexion strains.

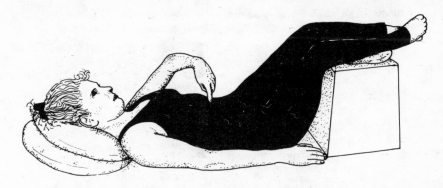

1st lumbar flexion strain. Contact tender point and vary degree of flexion — curling up — with rotation of knees to one side or other until tenderness abates — hold for 90 seconds

Lie on the back with cushions under the upper back and head as well as under the buttocks. The knees are flexed and supported, ideally by a helper but if not available then on a stool or seat of a chair.

For 1st lumbar flexion strains the tender point may be in (a) the region of the tip of the most prominent anterior (front) pelvic bone (near the point for 12th thoracic flexion strain) or (b) an inch or two towards the midline from (a).

Positioning for both of these points involves the general flexed (i.e. curled up) position described above, together with rotation and sidebending towards the side of the tender points, until sensitivity in the tender point is markedly lessened. Rotation and sidebending are achieved by ankles crossed for rotation.

This position does not require assistance. Maintain for 90 seconds.

For 2nd lumbar flexion strains there are also two possible tender points. The first (a)

is an inch or so more to the side from the tip of the prominent anterior pelvic bone or (b) 2 inches to the side of, and level with the navel.

Treatment of (a) involves the same flexed general position and movement of the pelvis. This involves marked rotation, and some sidebending of the pelvis away from the side of pain. Treatment of (b) involves the same general position and marked pelvic rotation towards the side of pain, together with some sidebending.

The 3rd lumbar flexion strain tender point is found half an inch below a line from L1(a) and L2(a).

The 4th lumbar flexion strain tender point is found in the groin where the ligament joins the pelvic bone.

The 5th lumbar flexion strain tender point is on the pubic bone near the centre.

These three (L3, 4, 5) all require flexion and sidebending which may be towards or away from the side of pain when fine tuning. L5 usually involves sidebending towards the side of pain.

Ample cushioning and some assistance make these procedures far easier. A great deal of patience may also be required to find the maximum position of ease.

Extension strains of the lumbar spine

The tender points for **1st and 2nd lumbar** extension (backwardbending) strains are found close to the tips of the transverse processes of the respective vertebrae, about 2½ inches from the midline. The position of ease for these is achieved by sidelying with the painful side uppermost.

The upper leg is allowed to come backwards to introduce extension into the low back. The leg is then allowed to fall towards the couch in a sort of scissors movement with the other leg.

Fine tuning is achieved by assessing sensitivity in the tender point. A helper is needed to maintain pressure here ideally, although self-monitoring is possible. The leg is taken into more or less extension backwards from the body.

The tender points for **3rd and 4th lumbar** extension strains are found on the crest of the pelvic bone, respectively about 3 inches and 5 inches lateral to the bony prominence, close to the base of the spine, where the crest of the pelvis ends.

Treatment may be achieved in the side-lying position, with the painful side uppermost and the upper leg extended behind the body. Unlike the method used for L1 and L2, the leg is raised from the couch into a degree of elevation (abduction).

This position requires assistance or adequate support, such as a stool or other firm support of the correct thickness.

In this position of backward excursion and elevation whilst in the sidelying position, the foot of this leg is rotated externally for fine tuning. However, it is impossible for this method to be self-administered without being a contortionist.

If performed in a face-down position, the leg can be elevated on a cushion and positioned so that it has been taken away from the midline sufficiently to reduce the sensitivity in the tender point, and external (outwards) rotation of the foot can then be used for fine tuning.

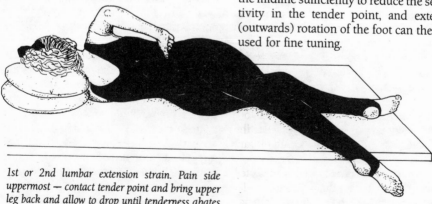

1st or 2nd lumbar extension strain. Pain side uppermost — contact tender point and bring upper leg back and allow to drop until tenderness abates — support and hold for 90 seconds

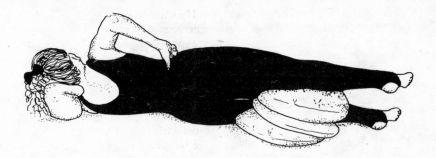

3rd-4th lumbar extension strain. Upper leg is elevated and supported by cushions — it is also brought backwards of body and some rotation of foot is introduced until tenderness in points abates — hold for 90 seconds.

There are three possible sites for extension strain of the last **(5th) lumbar vertebrae.**

(a) is between the spinous process of the last vertebrae and the sacrum.

(b) is on the superior surface of the sacrum.

(c) is located centrally on the sacrum.

Treatment of (a) and (c) is as for treatment of 1st and 2nd lumbar, as described above.

Treatment of (b) requires assistance. Lying on the unaffected side, the lower arm is allowed to hang over the side of the couch. The upper leg on the affected side is flexed and the helper supports the knee. This leg is taken more towards the head or the foot of the table, and elevated or depressed to the ceiling or the floor for fine tuning of pain relief in the tender point.

For any joint pain or strain it is suggested that you search the local muscles for tender areas, especially in the muscles which may have shortened during or after the strain.

As an example, let us think of a *sprained ankle* in which the foot 'turned' over, thus stretching the muscles on the outer aspect of the ankle. It is in these muscles that pain will be felt most strongly, but it is in the muscles which were not stretched during the strain, in fact in the ones which were if anything shortened during the strain on the inner aspect of the ankle, where the tender point relating to this strain will be found. If these non-painful tissues are probed by finger or thumb a localized sensitive area will be found. By maintaining pressure on it and positioning the ankle so that the tenderness vanishes from the point, a counterstrain situation will be achieved, which will often exaggerate the position in which the strain took place.

Having found this position and maintained it for 90 seconds the general pain in the joint should be much reduced. Of course, if actual tissue damage such as tearing or over-stretching occurred, this will still require time to heal.

By no means all joint strains and dysfunctions can be self-treated. However, a few are readily amenable to assistance by self-help or with assistance from a helper.

Use these methods for dealing with minor strains.

If there is only temporary relief seek professional advice.

These methods are not meant to take the place of expert treatment but are self-help, first-aid measures of supreme safety.

These include:

Shoulder problems in which there is pain and restriction.

These can often be eased by the following procedure if a tender point is found in the front of the joint and/or under it at the front of the axilla (arm-pit).

Sit in front of a low table with the elbow of the affected side resting on a pad on the table, and the upper arm held close to the chest.

Lean on to this to push the shoulder towards your ear until a position of relief is found.

Hold for 90 seconds.

Where the **biceps muscle insertion** is involved in **shoulder and upper arm** pain the tender point should be found below the collar bone in the soft tissues of the front of the shoulder.

Position of ease for tenderness in such points, involves lying face upwards with the upper arm flexed upwards with the lower arm also flexed and pointing in a direction somewhere between your head and directly backwards. Fine tuning involves taking the elbow more or less inwards or outwards and slightly altering the degree of elevation of the arm. Slight rotation of the upper arm may also be used to fine tune until pain is removed.

Tender points may also be found at the back of the joint, anywhere from the base of the neck across to the tip of the shoulder or in the muscles overlying the shoulder blade.

Experimentation as to the best position of ease is required and a search for this should be performed slowly.

If a helper is available, then the treatment position of lying face downwards would be better for points near the arm pit, behind the joint or behind the very tip of the joint. The arm is taken outwards and backwards, or backwards and across the body, both with variable degrees of rotation of the arm used to produce ease in tender points.

Self-treatment in these positions is difficult because of the complexity of maintaining contact with the tender point whilst at the same time manoeuvring the arm into a position of ease which is sustainable for 90 seconds.

Elbow tender points
These will be found anywhere from directly in front of the joint to areas at the side or behind the joint (depending upon just what strain has occurred). Positions of ease require diligent experimentation, varying from full flexion to complete extension (straight arm), all with variations on rotation of the lower arm, with the tender point providing the information as to the position of greatest ease.

Similar guides are suggested for the tender points found on the wrist and various surfaces of the hand relating to the many joints which may be strained or in pain in this region.

Knee dysfunction

The various tender points related to the associated strains will be found on the inner, outer or posterior surface, as well as under and around the knee-cap itself. Positions for relief of tender points may involve sitting or lying, knee flexed.

For tender points on the inner (medial) surface, the knee is flexed to around 60° and the lower leg is rotated outwards until relief is felt from sensitivity in the tender point. Hold for 90 seconds.

For tender points on the outer surface of the knee, the lateral surface, internal rotation of the lower leg is needed with the knee slightly flexed. Neither of these knee manoeuvres is easy to accomplish without assistance from a helper.

Tender point pain found behind the knee probably relates to (a) the posterior cruciate ligament, the tender point central on the knee crease or (b) to the anterior cruciate ligament, just above the knee crease slightly to the inner or outer side of the midline, or (c) to points found below the knee crease to either side, which seem to relate to strain of the gastrocnemius muscle.

The release of these involves, for (a) placing a pillow under the upper end of the large bone of the lower leg, the tibia, and having the helper push downwards on the lower aspect of the upper leg, just above the knee. At the same time, the foot is turned inwards. This combination of forces reduces the tender point activity and should be held for 90 seconds.

For (b) the pillow is placed under the lower end of the thigh, above the knee crease. The helper presses down on the upper aspect of the lower leg just below the knee. At the same time the lower leg is turned inwards until the tender point sensitivity is reduced. Hold for 90 seconds.

Since the helper will need two hands for these two manoeuvres, the patient needs to palpate the tender point all the while to ensure that sensitivity remains reduced throughout the procedure.

For (c) the leg is held straight and the toes strongly pointed downwards, (hyperextension of the ankle) until relief of sensitivity in the tender point is noted. Again hold for 90 seconds.

Tender points found on the front of the knee may relate to tendon or meniscus problems and require variations in procedure including:

1. Full extension of the knee (as straight as possible and pushing backwards) with the lower leg rotated inwards is required for patellar tendon tender point relief, this being found directly below the knee cap.

2. For dysfunction of the inner meniscus tender point, which lies on the inner aspect of the knee towards the lower edge of the patella, the helper takes the leg of the patient who is lying face upwards, lateral at the hip, and bracing the knee and at the same time monitoring the tender point with one hand, uses the other hand to rotate it inwards and to push the lower leg towards the midline without allowing the knee or the upper leg to move. This localizes the forces at the meniscus in question, reducing the tenderness.

3. For a tender point on the lateral meniscus found on the outer surface of the joint, the forces are opposite to the previous manoeuvre. The helper takes the leg outwards (abduction) and braces the knee,

monitoring the tender point with one hand. The other hand is used to take the lower leg outwards at the knee and to rotate it outwards, until the sensitivity reduces in the tenderpoint.

A variety of positions are available for dealing with the multitude of tender points found on the foot, relating to ankle strain or to other joints of the foot.

Self-treatment in this region is easy and a combination of Strain/counterstrain and Muscle Energy Technique can be used to relieve most joint problems in the region to some extent, often completely.

Use tender points to assist in finding ways of easing pain in this manner even if they are of long standing.

It will certainly be found that Strain/counterstrain methods are more suited to recent injuries, especially if spasm is a feature, for example with whiplash injuries, but some relief is to be gained for even chronic problems, which may then benefit from other methods such as Muscle Energy Technique.

Whether a joint problem is spinal or involves a small joint anywhere else, the marvellous discoveries of Lawrence Jones can be used to ease discomfort and release spasm via this totally painless and uniquely safe system.

Index